The Lost Soul Companion

The Lost Soul

A book of
Comfort and Constructive
Advice for Black Sheep,
Square Pegs, Struggling Artists,
and Other Free Spirits

Companion

Susan M. Brackney

A Dell Book

A Dell Trade Paperback
Published by
Dell Publishing
a division of
Random House, Inc.
1540 Broadway
New York, New York 10036

Copyright © 1999 by Susan M. Brackney
Book design by *O'Lanso Gabbidon*
For permission credits and copyright notices, see page 157–159.

Reprinted by arrangement with Puckitt Press, Inc.

DTP and the colophon are trademarks of Random House, Inc.

ISBN: 0-440-50921-1

Library of Congress Catalog Card Number: 99-091690

Printed in the United States of America

Published simultaneously in Canada

September 2001

10   9   8   7   6   5   4   3   2   1
FFG

For you.

acknowledgments

How can I ever thank you enough?

* Mom and Dad for teaching me that a ship in port is safe but it never goes anywhere!

* Brother and Leann for their general encouragement and help with the light bulb contraption...

* Peter... for EVERYTHING !!

* Jeff Rosenplot for his moral support, ability to motivate, and fantastic design skills... he designed my first edition!!

* Martina Gray for taking many of the photos you see here...

* Eric White for still more technical support...

* also thank you to all of my interviewees — especially the shy ones.

* For their help with my research, thank you to Temple Grandin, Dalt Wonk, Danny Gamble, and the research librarians at the Monroe County Public Library...

* Michael White, Michael Teague, Jennifer, Amy, Andrew, and all of my other editors... thank you so much!

* VALDA and Marianne for their encouragement and understanding.

* Rick for his kind words and good suggestions for "Things to Do Instead of Killing Yourself"

* Stephanie for her companionship and good ideas...

* Wes for the fantastic paper plate story and taking me to Burning Man...

* Kevin Greenlee and Melissa Gray for setting me straight on a few things!

* Andrea Scher, Debra Goldstein, Jamie Ehrlich, and Kathleen Jayes for their generosity and vision...

and God, Dr. Barnes, and the makers of Zoloft.

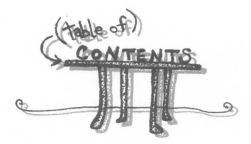

III. CREATIVE COPING

IV. LIVING WELL

Eleven Thoughtful Letters and My Wildest Expectations

A while ago I wrote and self-published this very book. My goals back then were to help as many people as I could and maybe to break even financially. I didn't quite break even on my own, but I *do* know that I've helped people because so far I've received eleven thoughtful letters from complete strangers thanking me for having written *The Lost Soul Companion.* They were the kind of letters that most people never get in their whole lives, and I got eleven! I know that my book made a difference to some people and that's very important to me.

As if getting nice letters wasn't enough, things became downright surreal when Dell, a division of Random House, decided to reprint *The Lost Soul Companion.* Certainly, that exceeded my wildest expectations! I am thankful that, with their help, more people will have access to my little book. What follows is *The Lost Soul Companion* just as it was meant to be. If you are a Lost—or even a Not-So-Lost—Soul, I hope you will find inspiration in these pages.

Yours,
Susan

The Lost Soul Companion

WHO ARE THE LOST SOULS?

I remember riding around at night with my parents in our little blue Volkswagen Rabbit. I was just a little girl and I loved looking into the windows of people's houses as we drove by.

Winter was an especially good time for this because the leaves were off the trees and families gathered indoors much earlier than usual. I would glimpse people eating dinner or washing their dishes or relaxing in front of their TVs—sometimes I could even see what they were watching, but only for a second and then it was on to the next house. A whole neighborhood at thirty miles an hour looked something like: dinner——television——dinner—— dark——dishes——dinner——dark——dark——dark.

I was a voyeur at age five. I could tell you it was the contrast of the warm, bright houses against the nighttime that attracted me, but that's not the whole truth. Those night drives reinforced my feeling of not belonging anywhere—

a feeling I didn't really mind. At twenty-seven, I'm still a detached but keenly interested observer. I still don't feel that I belong anywhere and I still don't mind the not be-longing—at least not much. I'm a Lost Soul.

If you've managed to find this obscure little book and it speaks to you, odds are good that you, too, are a Lost Soul. You already know that being a Lost Soul is something of a mixed blessing.

Lost Souls are highly creative and all too often prone to fits of lethargy and despair. (For my part, I've battled severe clinical depression since 1990. With medication and ther-apy, I've been able to manage a relatively stable existence.)

Sometimes we feel disconnected, but the good news is that we are actually in very good company.

Lost Souls are struggling artists, musicians, actors, writ-ers—in short, those people taking the road less traveled. It may have made all the difference to Robert Frost, but that particular path can make its wanderers feel very alone. We may feel like black sheep, failures, or unwelcome guests, but we don't have to.

I've learned a good deal about the pitfalls of the "starv-ing artist" lifestyle and I hope that you'll get some good from my mistakes. In 1997, believing that geography was my only obstacle, I moved 2,000 miles away from my friends and family in order to better pursue my art career (and to be with my boyfriend at the time . . .).

I lasted only a couple of months in Santa Cruz, California, and I'd spent all of my savings there just to survive. I became suicidal. I left many of my belongings behind and took an emergency flight home.

Back home in Indiana, I felt like a failure. I began to wonder if any other people felt as hopeless as I did. I had so many big ideas but I couldn't even get out of bed. I wanted to know other Lost Souls. I thought if only we could compare notes I might not feel so hopeless and uninspired.

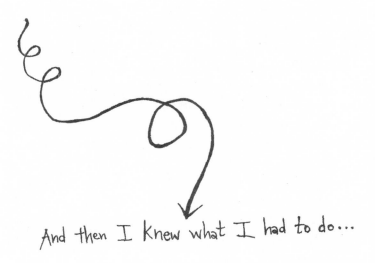

And then I knew what I had to do...

I AM HERE . . .
WHERE ARE YOU?

Eight years ago I heard a
biology professor speak about
migratory songbirds. He said that
most birds out in the wild use "phatic
communication." This kind of communication
isn't about specific infor-
mation; rather, it's about
sharing feelings and
establishing a mood of sociabil-
ity and community. In other words,
if you see two birds' little feathered
breasts heaving with effort, endlessly
chirping back and forth to one another, the
exchange might be translated like this:

i am here...Where are you?

Bird #1: I am here . . . where are you?

Bird #2: I'm here . . . where are you?

And so on and so on and so on. Maybe this is reassuring for them; it was very reassuring for me to know that I'm not the only creature in the world who does this sort of thing.

   The Lost Soul Companion is really just me perched high on my branch, standing on one leg, singing, "I am here . . . where are you?"

What Is *The Lost Soul Companion*?

On the surface, *The Lost Soul Companion* is my little bit of phatic communication. But, with the involvement of other Lost Souls, it can breathe on its own.

The Lost Soul Companion can also be found at www.lostsoulcompanion.com on the World Wide Web. My hope is that the site will serve as an ongoing appendix to this book. In addition, visiting Lost Souls may post comments, questions, and encouraging messages for one another.

A *Lost Soul Companion* pen pal program may also be in the works. . . .

Finally, Lost Souls are encouraged to submit original poetry, artwork, essays, etc., for the benefit of other website visitors.

I hope that both the printed and web versions of *The Lost Soul Companion* will foster a sense of community for struggling artists of all kinds. I want us to be better equipped to deal with life's disappointments and more motivated, productive, and better prepared for success as well.

ONE MORE THING . . .

An old friend, after reading an early draft of *The Lost Soul Companion,* said, "The whole thing seems pretty arrogant if you ask me. Who do you think you are to write this book?"

It's true that I'm very young and my experience is still rather limited. I began to wonder if I should scrap the whole project. After all, isn't it awfully presumptuous of me to think that I have something of value to say to you? Well, perhaps . . . But if I can help even one Lost Soul to feel more connected and hopeful, then I'll risk seeming presumptuous.

Who do you think you are?

1.

Misery,
Suicide

&

Hothouse
Flowers

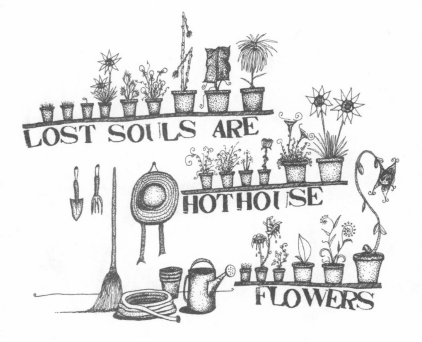

LOST SOULS ARE HOTHOUSE FLOWERS

Lost Souls Are Hothouse Flowers

L ost Souls are hothouse flowers—delicate, beautiful, fragile, and rare. Some require special attention. Some like to be left alone. Some thrive with lots of light while others prefer darkness. They are all very different and spectacular in their own ways.

There are droopy, weeping plants prone to fits of trembling (*Dangley biticus-tremulus*).

Some are afraid to grow at all (*Timidus minitus*) and others just can't get properly motivated despite their best intentions to flower (*Perhapsus laterum*).

Some plants are continually sick with some fungus or another (*Ickacus neglectum*).

There is the *Supra egosimo,* which grows in uneven, angry bursts. If conditions are not exactly to its specifications, it releases a very foul odor.

There are self-destructive plants whose thorns turn inward, piercing the plants' very stems (*I. Destructus*).

Some of the plants can only grow when throngs of people coo appreciatively at them. If they are not properly admired very regularly, they will die (*Externita needeveria*).

I have been all of these flowers at one time or another. Most often I am the *Shaded melancholanata,* which grows as best as it can inside a dark, zippered bag. Very few people have actually seen its flowers although they are rumored to be breathtaking. No one knows why it has become accustomed to the darkness; perhaps it was just always so.

It is important to note that all of these unusual plants do cross-pollinate. As a result, there are hothouses full of

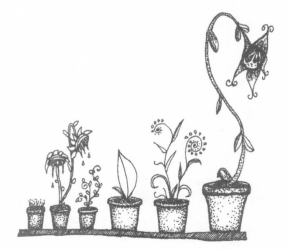

incomprehensible variations. Truly, there are too many to describe. They are challenging to tend to, but their potential for beauty is unlimited. With proper care, some of the most hopeless varieties offer velvety leaves, ethereal perfumes, and blossoms so rich with color they very nearly hum.

Which kind are you?

HEY!

Just in case you skipped the introduction (I almost always do!), I'll say again that I want Lost Souls to be better equipped to deal with Life's disappointments and more motivated, productive, and better prepared for success as well. But before we can get to the business of living well, we have to address the misery and suicidal tendencies which sometimes plague us...

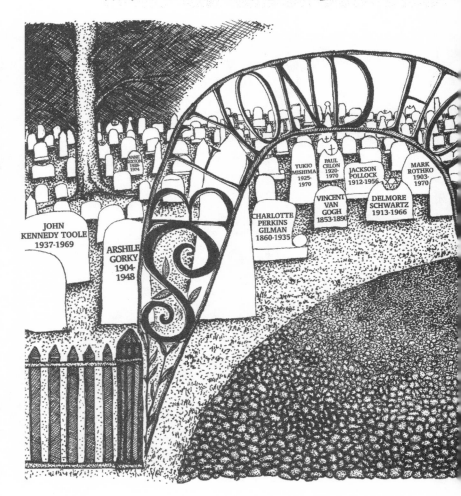

JOHN KENNEDY TOOLE 1937-1969

ARSHILE GORKY 1904 1948

ANNE SEXTON 1928-1974

CHARLOTTE PERKINS GILMAN 1860-1935

YUKIO MISHIMA 1925-1970

PAUL CELON 1920-1970

JACKSON POLLOCK 1912-1956

VINCENT VAN GOGH 1853-1890

DELMORE SCHWARTZ 1913-1966

MARK ROTHKO 1903-1970

didn't handle Life's difficulties well enough...

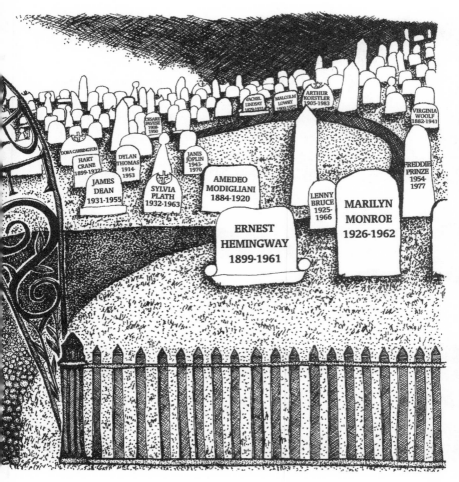

LOST SOULS AND SUICIDE

I've thought about killing myself many times. Maybe you have too. Hopefully I can convince us both that it's not such a good idea.

For years, so-called "experts" have said that even the mention of suicide to someone who is himself suicidal is tantamount to pushing him off a ledge or helping him pull the trigger. I don't believe that.

Having suicidal feelings from time to time is common. It's crucial to talk about our feelings of hopelessness and desperation because there is no reason we have to go on feeling this way. If you share your darkest thoughts with other Lost Souls, you'll find comfort in your similarities.

I've known for years that I'm not all here. Many creative types aren't. According to *Science News* (May 1994), a Harvard Medical School psychiatrist conducted a study which concluded that "Artists suffer more than their share of depression, a tendency that may fuel their creativity while it shatters their personal lives."

Many of our most cherished writers, artists, musicians, and poets have fallen victim to what has been called "excessive sensitivity." In his work *The Savage God: A Study of Suicide,* A. Alvarez writes, "The casualty rate among the gifted seems all out of proportion, as though the nature of the artistic undertaking itself and the demands it makes

had altered radically [during the twentieth century]."
When Lost Souls suffer enough emotional pain, suicide
becomes a tempting—and permanent—solution to every
problem. Every Lost Soul on pages 16 and 17 chose to
"solve" their problems this way. Add in the tendency to
glorify and romanticize the act, and suicide's appeal grows
again.

In 1955 actor James Dean was only twenty-four when
he slammed his Porsche into another car and died instantly.
It's widely believed that his "accident" was intentional, and
I used to think this crash was just another garden-variety
suicide. I may have been wrong about that, though.

Wrong because James Dean's mechanic was with him in
the car that day. If this was a suicide attempt, wouldn't
that mean Dean had no regard for the life of his mechanic?
It's possible, I guess, since suicidal people often lack regard
for the lives they leave behind, but we'll never really know.

Let's say James Dean *had* lived through his car accident
(and some people actually believe this, by the way), I suspect that it wouldn't have been long before Death collected
him in a bar fight, a drug overdose, or something else.
Rather than suggesting this was an outright suicide, it is
safer to say that James Dean was a "chronic suicide" instead.
Chronic suicides are people who live very reckless lives because they actually *want* to die.

In death, Dean is glamorized, but in life he was, not to put too fine a point on it, something of an asshole. He abused alcohol and other drugs and had an explosive temper. It has been over forty-five years since his death and James Dean still gets fan mail.

If you ask me, those fans are wasting their stamps and their time. Dead is forever and, as far as I know, James Dean isn't reading his mail. Right now he's just a pile of bones in a box in a hole in Fairmont, Indiana. How glamorous.

FAMOUS SUICIDES AND WHAT-IFS . . .

VINCENT AND THEO VAN GOGH

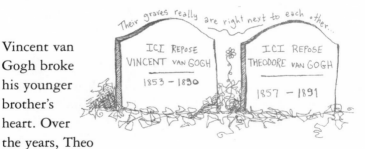

Their graves really are right next to each other...

ICI REPOSE
VINCENT VAN GOGH
1853 – 1890

ICI REPOSE
THEODORE VAN GOGH
1857 – 1891

Vincent van Gogh broke his younger brother's heart. Over the years, Theo van Gogh supported Vincent financially and emotionally despite his own frailties and commitments. He adored Vincent and did everything in his power to further his brother's art and his independence. Vincent had a long history of madness and, despite his brother's efforts, he shot himself in the chest on July 27, 1890. He died two days later. Just three months after Vincent's suicide, Theo, beside himself with grief, completely broke down. On January 25, 1891, he died in an asylum. According to Jan Hulsker's book *Vincent and Theo van Gogh: A Dual Biography,* "In a lecture published by the Kröller-Müller Foundation in 1954, these words were devoted to Theo's illness and death: 'The doctor who treated him with great devotion, tried in vain to get his attention by reading to him an article . . . about Vincent. The only interest he had was for the name Vincent. In the "history of illness" it says in the column "cause of disease: chronic illness, excessive exertion and sorrow." ' " Vincent's selfish act had major repercussions on other lives.

SYLVIA PLATH

On February 11, 1963, Sylvia Plath took milk and a plate of bread upstairs to her two children, Frieda and Nicholas. Then she returned to the kitchen, sealed the window and the door, and stuck her head in the gas oven. It was the last in a succession of suicide attempts. This one worked.

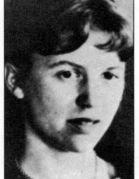

AP/Wide World Photo

It was only a month after the publication of her critically acclaimed work *The Bell Jar.* Despite great successes throughout her life, Sylvia was plagued with self-doubt and bouts of serious depression. Occasionally she sought treatment for these episodes. Hospitalization, electric shock therapy, and psychiatric treatment were helpful, but it's important to note that really effective antidepressant medications weren't yet available.

A. Alvarez, a friend to Sylvia, doesn't believe she actually wanted to die. Alvarez maintains that this suicide attempt was just another cry for help in a long series. It is an especially likely prospect since, as he explains in *The Savage God,* the au pair girl who found Sylvia's body also found a note saying "Please call Dr.———," and giving his telephone number. He writes, "This time . . . there was too much holding her to life. Above all, there were the children: she was too passionate a mother to want to lose them or them to lose her." But her crying wolf lost those children the most important person in their lives.

VIRGINIA WOOLF

On March 28, 1941, Virginia Woolf placed a large stone in her pocket and walked into the River Ouse in Sussex, England. It was widely believed that her suicide was related to her distress over World War II, but that was not the case. The true cause is revealed to her husband, Leonard, in her suicide note:

I have the feeling I shall go mad. I hear voices and cannot concentrate on my work. I have fought against it, but cannot fight any longer. You have been so perfectly good. I cannot go on and spoil your life.

Virginia Woolf's life had been riddled with illness and nervous breakdowns. Scholars believe that she feared this latest episode would be permanent. Leonard Woolf had been "perfectly good" to his wife. He cared for her during her illnesses and did his best to prevent future breakdowns, but, clearly, Virginia felt guilty for requiring so much care and attention. I imagine, however, that her husband was happy to comfort her and would have preferred that she live. Her assumption of her own lack of worth took away Leonard's ability to help her.

The list of famous suicides goes on for miles. They left loved ones behind to grieve for them and much unfinished business to do. I understand that sometimes the love of

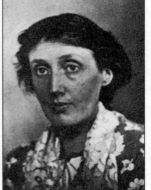

23

friends and family doesn't seem like enough in the face of so much pain. For me, the urge to die has been powerful, but the thought of leaving my mother and father behind to suffer such a loss keeps me hanging on by my fingernails.

These Lost Souls were hurting, but that doesn't excuse their actions—especially in light of the fact that depression and other mental disorders were somewhat treatable at the time, and now much more so. No one in the throes of despair is thinking clearly. That's why it's so important to ask someone else for help.

I wonder what could have been if they had chosen to live. What incredible works of art have we missed out on because they chose to die? Sylvia Plath would be in her sixties today. Maybe she would still be writing. There are songs we'll never get to hear, paintings we'll never see, novels we can't enjoy because their creators gave up.

Living is really hard, but death is forever. We're all going to die eventually, so what's your rush? Even if you think committing suicide will make you seem tragic and romantic and cool, you'll never know what happened anyway. Don't you want to know how your life was supposed to turn out? Wouldn't you like to see what you're made of?

Dorothy Parker said it all best
with her poem

Resume

Razors pain you;
Rivers are damp;
Acids stain you;
And drugs cause cramp.
Guns aren't lawful;
Nooses give;
Gas smells awful;
You might as well live.

25

JOHN KENNEDY TOOLE

When I told my friend Stephanie about *The Lost Soul Companion* project, she told me about John Kennedy Toole. He wrote her favorite book, *A Confederacy of Dunces*—a fantastically funny novel about a guy named Ignatius Reilly and his adventures in New Orleans. The work won Toole the Pulitzer Prize, but he didn't live to see his success. Instead he died thinking he was an utter failure. I wish I could bring him back from the dead and show him what a contribution he made, but I can't.

Ken Toole was born in New Orleans in 1937. Throughout his life he was very close to his mother, Thelma, who fostered in her son a love for learning and "high culture." Ken was an unusually gifted child with an I.Q. of 133 as a first grader. He graduated from high school at age sixteen. At twenty he graduated from Tulane with honors in English and a Woodrow Wilson Fellowship for graduate studies. In 1957 he matriculated at Columbia University, where he completed a two-year master's literature program in just one year. He was a literature professor at Hunter College in Manhattan and then a faculty member at the University of Southwestern Louisiana until 1961, when he was drafted. In the army, he taught English at Fort Buchanan, Puerto Rico. Surprisingly, his position afforded him his own private quarters and plenty of time to write.

A Confederacy of Dunces resulted. After his discharge, Ken returned to New Orleans and immediately submitted his manuscript to Simon & Schuster for publication. Soon after, the publishing house sent a letter which was so encouraging that publication seemed imminent. But, according to New Orleans writer Dalt Wonk, the letter was merely the first in a disappointing series. In his two-part work "John Kennedy Toole's Odyssey Among the Dunces," Wonk described the events:

> *Over the next few months, other letters arrived from Simon & Schuster. Thelma knew because she usually picked up the mail. But Ken did not show them to her. "He wanted to spare me," she said later, "for he knew they would grieve me."*
>
> *It was only after her son's death that Thelma was to read the correspondence.*
>
> *Robert Gottlieb, an editor with the publishing house, wanted extensive revisions, she said.*
>
> *Thelma would hear Ken typing by the hour in his room.*
>
> *As the months passed, Thelma says, the requests for changes continued.*
>
> *Ken became frantic. His opportunity was fading. Thelma says his letters to Gottlieb took on a beseeching tone.*
>
> *"My son got down on his knees and begged. He humbled*

himself before that man. He told Gottlieb he had poured his soul into the book."

Wonk continued: "After two years of dickering, Thelma says, Gottlieb rejected the book."

Ultimately, Ken gave up the search for a publisher. On January 20, 1969, he began a two-month-long journey. He drove to California, then Georgia—stopping to see the Hearst Mansion and the home of Flannery O'Connor—and, finally, to a wooded area in Biloxi, Mississippi, where he ran a garden hose from his tailpipe to one of his back windows. Three boys discovered his body. The car's engine was still running.

Until recently, there was a tendency to blame the publishing industry for his death. Joel Fletcher was one of Ken Toole's friends and has written a memoir about Ken and Thelma. Fletcher explained, "Robert Gottlieb has pretty much taken a bum rap in the story of Ken and *Confederacy*. The version that is 'out there' is Thelma's much simplified and grossly

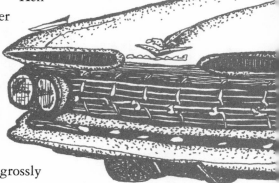

unfair version. . . . Suffice it to say, there were really no villains in this story, only victims."

Some scholars now suggest that Ken Toole's disappointment was compounded by many other problems including his domineering mother, financial burdens, binge drinking, questions about his sexuality, and, as if those weren't enough, the early signs of what might have been schizophrenia.

After his death, Thelma Toole decided to continue the search for a publisher.

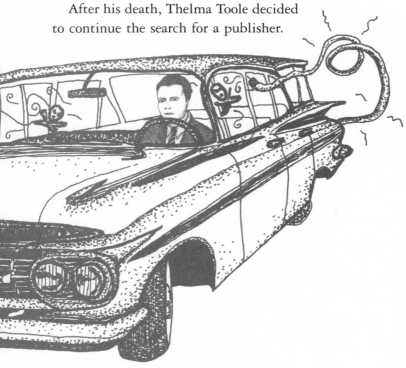

She succeeded nearly nine years later—thanks to the help of Walker Percy, an influential local novelist. In 1980, Louisiana State University published *A Confederacy of Dunces,* and it won the Pulitzer Prize. Ken Toole left another novel, *The Neon Bible,* behind, but, had he lived, what else could he have offered us? I'm deeply saddened when I think of the body of work that died with John Kennedy Toole, and I know that things didn't have to turn out this way.

I wish Ken Toole had had the support he needed back then, and, if I had known him, I would've tried to encourage less traditional thinking—at least with regard to the publishing industry.

There's something to be said for starting out small. Although he might not have wanted to, Ken Toole could've self-published. It's not nearly as glamorous, but if all he really wanted was to see his work in print and in the hands of his readers, it would have been a perfectly acceptable solution. If, on the other hand, he desired the financial success and notoriety that sometimes come with being published by a large, established company such as Simon & Schuster, I would not have been of much help.

I can't support any plan which relies too heavily on the fickle world of publishing. Ken Toole was brilliant, but he made the mistake of pinning his hopes on an industry in which luck and connections are often more important than talent.

In case you haven't yet come across the part where I tell you that you won't always get what you need, allow me to say it again. You really won't always get what you need—or what you think you need—from the rest of the world. It's best to accept this reality and learn to depend on yourself.

Now all that's left to do is appreciate his work and try to learn from his mistakes. Like John Kennedy Toole, you can be brilliant, motivated, and productive, but, please, do leave the giving-up part behind. After all, garden hoses are for watering things and there is plenty of despair around as it is.

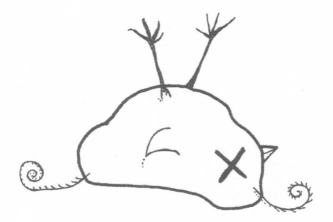

2.

Having Hope,

Getting Motivated

Being Strong

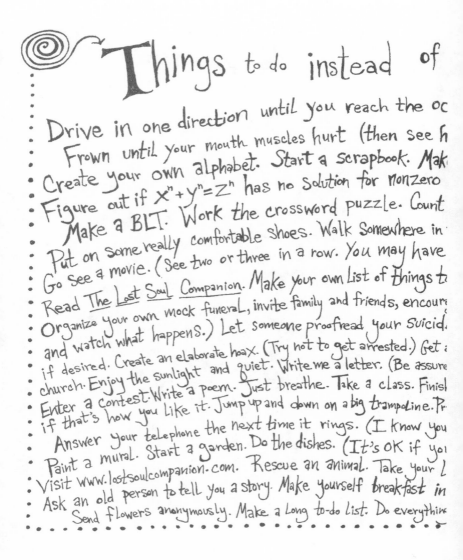

Things to do instead of

Drive in one direction until you reach the oc

Frown until your mouth muscles hurt (then see h

Create your own alphabet. Start a scrapbook. Mak

Figure out if $x^n + y^n = z^n$ has no solution for nonzero

Make a BLT. Work the crossword puzzle. Count

Put on some really comfortable shoes. Walk somewhere in

Go see a movie. (See two or three in a row. You may have

Read The Lost Soul Companion. Make your own list of things t

Organize your own mock funeral, invite family and friends, encour

and watch what happens.) Let someone proofread your suicid

if desired. Create an elaborate hoax. (Try not to get arrested.) Get

church. Enjoy the sunlight and quiet. Write me a letter. (Be assure

Enter a contest. Write a poem. Just breathe. Take a class. Finish

if that's how you like it. Jump up and down on a big trampoline. Pr

Answer your telephone the next time it rings. (I know you

Paint a mural. Start a garden. Do the dishes. (It's OK if yo

Visit www.lostsoulcompanion.com. Rescue an animal. Take your L

Ask an old person to tell you a story. Make yourself breakfast in

Send flowers anonymously. Make a long to-do list. Do everythin

Killing Yourself... ←

:ean. Say hello to everyone you pass during the day.
low much easier it is to smile.)
e something you invented or invent something you can make.
integers x,y, and z if n is an integer greater than two.
backwards from 10 billion by 13s. Visit a yard sale.
them. Make something nice for someone – give it to them.
to make extended visits to the restroom between films.)
o do instead of killing yourself (and then do them.)
age them to eulogize you. (Tell them how you've really been feeling
e note. Build a fort. Meditate. Shampoo your hair... repeat
arrested. Blow the stink off! (See page 117.) Sneak into a
ed of a hopeful reply.) Volunteer somewhere. Doodle.
h something you started. Drink a cup of tea with sugar and milk...
ay. Eat a tomato. Pet a kitty cat. Smoke a cigarette. (It's slower.)
i haven't been...) Ask a stranger for some good advice.
u've let them pile up. Wash a couple of them at least.)
oose change to the bank. Play some beautiful music.
bed. Eat cookies. Stare at clouds. Visit the maternity ward.
g on it. Set a world record. Open the curtains.

Do Something . . . Anything!

Anthony Storr, in his essay "The Darkness That Has Brought Humanity Light," writes, "Many of the most valuable human beings who have ever lived have shown clear evidence of recurrent depression. What matters is that those who exhibit this liability should be able to use it productively." In addition to regular therapy and, in some cases, medication, doing something—anything— is better than doing nothing when you feel terrible. When I am in my darkest place, simply getting out of bed is tantamount to moving a mountain with a teaspoon. Getting started is the hardest part. It gets easier after that. I promise.

CREATIVITY AND DEPRESSION: GETTING OUT OF THE HOLE

There's no doubt in my mind that without the love of my parents, support of great counselors, and access to the antidepressant drug Zoloft, I would be dead now. I drew this self-portrait in the initial stages of my bout with panic disorder and depression back in 1988.

I remember showing it to my mother, who looked terribly disturbed when I told her that my brains were coming out of the top of my head. (She had hoped it was just a strangely knitted cap.)

I knew I couldn't expect to feel happy and wonderful all of the time, but mine were not ordinary ups and downs. At that time I was always physically exhausted. I had little or no appetite for food—or life for that matter. Nameless despair, fear, and hopelessness overwhelmed me. I cried all the time. Well-meaning friends and distant relatives told me to smile, to cheer up. That just made me feel worse. My parents knew better; they got me the medical attention I so desperately needed.

I don't know if my problems with depression are tied to the fact that I'm a creative person, but research suggests that creativity and mental illness—especially manic depression—are closely linked. The good news is that depressive illnesses are very responsive to treatment.

In my case, I went to my doctor and the psychologist my parents chose for me just to pacify them. I knew in my heart that I was a lost cause, that all the special treatment was a waste of their money. I felt terribly guilty about that especially. I couldn't remember a time when I didn't feel miserable. It was just my personality.

But a month or so into my treatment—I was seeing the psychologist a few times a week and had begun taking Zoloft—I was delighted to admit that I'd been wrong about everything. I was really starting to feel better. It was as if I'd been driving down an unfamiliar country road in the dark without my headlights, and suddenly they'd been flipped on. I could see where I was going and it didn't look half bad. (I should tell you, of course, that even with my medication, I still have some very bad weeks, but I get by.)

The doctors told me that some people have to stay on antidepressant medications their entire lives and others can take a short course of the drugs and then be done with them. It appears that I am among the first category. I've tried to taper off my medication and I've tried to stop taking it altogether, but each time I was right back where I started—in the hole.

I tell you this not to discourage you, but so you'll know that it really is possible to feel better—with help. There is seldom a quick fix, but, the good news is, there are ways to cope.

A Little More on Antidepressants

Some people argue that it is simply trendy to rely on mood-altering medications such as Prozac and that most antidepressant users need nothing more than a swift kick in the ass. Once in a while that swift kick in the ass business may have merit, but legitimate medical need for antidepressants shouldn't be discounted. The truth is antidepressants don't do much of anything for people who don't really need them. In other words, antidepressants don't make "normal" people feel happier but they do make depressed people feel more normal.

There are currently about 25 different antidepressants on the market and the very first ones were introduced in the 1950s and '60s. The older classes of antidepressants—the tricyclics and the monoamine oxidase inhibitors—aren't used nearly as frequently now. They have largely been replaced by selective serotonin reuptake inhibitors such as Serzone, Luvox, Paxil, Zoloft, and Prozac. Other kinds include Remeron, Effexor, Trazodone, and Wellbutrin.

These newer drug classes are very effective and their side effects aren't quite as bad as those of their predecessors.

The natural dietary supplement St. John's Wort shouldn't be overlooked as a potential relief, but as far as I can tell, trying to fight severe clinical depression with small doses of this medicinal herb is tantamount to spitting in the sea.

If you have a serious problem with depression, you _must_ see a doctor and discuss your options. Remember, there's hope even if you don't think so right now!

Too Many
Naps and the
Bad Day Box

When I take every-
thing and everyone
around me too seriously,
I make myself miserable.
Those are the days when I'm so
overwhelmed that I just want to bury
my head under the pillows and sleep my life away. I've
found that taking a five-hour nap is the next best thing to
suicide, because it's not as permanent a departure from
life's difficulties. (My family would be devastated if I actually killed myself. As it is, they're simply a little concerned
about my excessive napping.)

And even though this is not a very popular opinion in
artistic circles, it really is possible to take too many naps. I
used to get home from work around four, "rest my eyes"
until nine, and then wake up just long enough to prepare
for bed. Once tucked in, I would not stir until seven the
next morning. It was exhausting.

There was a long stretch of weeks when I was floating
into work on an enormous dark cloud. I put my dresses
on over my pajamas. My performance on the job was
mediocre to substandard at best. Valda, one of my

coworkers, must've noticed what a mess I had become because she made me the Bad Day Box. It made all the difference.

It was a paper cube with little hinged doors all over it. The one on top read "Bad Day Box—Pick a door as needed . . . Do not overdose." She had carefully glued tiny stars and moons all over the outside of the box. It was elaborate and lovely and I was energized just knowing that I had a Bad Day Box which had been created just for me.

Over the next few months, I peeked behind the doors—but only when it was completely necessary. There were whimsical illustrations and great suggestions to breathe a little life back into me. In case you're curious, here are the different doors:

The first door: "Eat Popcorn—Stand in the cafeteria and listen to it pop and smell it! Share it with someone!" was written alongside a red-and-white-striped bag bursting with popcorn.

The next door: "Take a walk outside, around the building, down by the stream, and then, turn around and walk around the other way!" was written spiraled around a sun.

The next: A giant, ringing telephone. "Turn your phone off for one hour—That's what voice mail is for!"

The one after that: "Go out to lunch with an old friend! Or call one and set a dinner date—so you'll have it to look forward to all day!"

The next to last: "Look at an old project you liked and remember that whatever you are doing now will soon be done and beautiful too!" A happy lady's giant face beamed from behind the message.

The very last door: A fluttery, long list. "Make a list of ten things you would do differently on a project—focus on how much better things will go next time and how much you learned!"

I confess that I didn't always obey the messages behind the doors. When Valda found that out, she nearly took my Bad Day Box away, but I convinced her to let me keep it. It did its job well. I took fewer naps. I decided to lighten up and do something for a change. Just think, if she hadn't have made me a Bad Day Box, I might still be asleep.

Now some marketing man with pointy elbows will snatch up Valda's Bad Day Box and mass produce them. There will be kits for crafty people with no imagination and even less dexterity. Don't buy those things. Try to make your own and give it to someone who really needs it.

Surrounding Ourselves

I'm one of the luckiest Lost Souls because I've managed to surround myself with supportive, kind people who are at least as stable as I am. When I feel especially lost, my tendency is to hide in my house and not come out. I don't eat. I don't answer the phone. I don't even go to the mailbox. That's where my friends and family come in.

On a few occasions they've let themselves into my house, helped clean me up, and get me back to "normal." I'm always happy to see them even though I may have been avoiding them all along. To really beat depression, avoiding isolation is essential. We may not want anyone around, but we can't survive without some kind of support system in place.

How to make friends: Be a friend. Don't look too hard. Be brave!
enjoy your own company even if you feel lonely.
go to bookstores, little cafes, art openings,
history lectures...
Have ADVENTURES with yourself!

→ If you think you are good company, others will too!

How to Make Your Very Own Snow Globe . . . and Why You Would Want to Do a Thing Like That

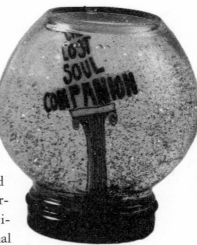

A side from surrounding yourself with good people, you might also try surrounding yourself with tangible reminders of your personal goals. What do you want for your life? What motivates you?

I've always liked the concept of the snow globe. (Who ever thought of it?) There's something very peaceful about watching glittery imitation snow swirling around a static scene—even if the scene itself leaves something to be desired. (I don't appreciate delicate figurines of small children or ice-skating teddy bears. For me, it's the snow inside the globe that does it.) As the snow sparkles down over everything, I just know it's really very quiet inside there. I want to climb in—not to be closer to the kitsch but, rather, to enjoy the stillness, the magic.

I saw homemade snow globes featured in an issue of *Martha Stewart Living* magazine. Until then, it had never occurred to me to try to make my own. They're very easy to make, and I've now made entirely too many of them. In each of my homemade snow globes I've substituted edgier subjects for the usual fare—subjects that mean much more to me than miniaturized, angel-faced Hummels.

You may decide that you too want to make your own snow globes. Just in case, here's how:

For starters you'll need a jar—baby food jars are a nice size but not necessarily a great shape. Poke around; I'm sure you'll find something suitable. You'll also need some enamel spray paint, epoxy, plastic glitter/snow, water, and glycerin. As for the scene inside your snow globe, choose glass, ceramic, or plastic figures and avoid wooden or metal objects as they will eventually become quite yucky. I discovered that the Shrinky Dinks of my youth work very well. Remember those? They were sheets of plastic you could draw on, color, cut out, and then bake in the oven for a minute. The oven's heat shrank the designs into much smaller, thicker versions—perfect, it turns out, for the insides of snow globes. I highly recommend them.

To get started, clean the jar well and remove the lid. Sand the jar lid inside and out, and paint the outside with enamel paint. Once the lid is completely dry, epoxy your subject or scene to the inside of the jar lid. Even though you may not want to wait, you really should allow the epoxy to set up overnight. Next, fill the jar almost to the top with water, add a pinch of plastic glitter/snow and a dash of glycerin (this helps prevent the snow from falling too quickly), and screw on the lid. (You may choose to line the lid with silicone or glue to prevent leaking.)

Now you should shake your snow globe, set it down on a table, sit back, and say, "What a hunk of shit!" At least that's what my friend Paul says. (He considers the whole project "mere dawdling.") Clearly, the snow globe project isn't for everyone. What may provide magic and inspiration for some people is nothing but a glittery horror to others. But I know there is hope in a good snow globe.

The scenes I've surrounded with snow and water illustrate my personal goals. There's the tiny house, the chickens, and dogs which I do not yet own. There's a trampoline full of friends. There are positive sayings (my battle cry: "She who dares, wins!"), uplifting reminders ("When one is always doing, it's amazing what one can do"), and whimsical creatures . . . just because.

I get a lot out of representing my goals and ideals in this way, but, in my more depressed moments, I feel cruelly taunted by so many unfulfilled desires encased in glass. On bad days I hide my snow globes, but I never have to hide them for very long.

THE PRECIPICE OF SUCCESS

The Precipice of Success is a giant, pointy mountain that looks like this:

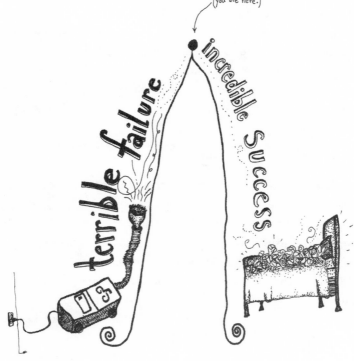

(you are here.)

terrible failure

incredible Success

The right side of the mountain offers great success, interviews on the *Today* show, a bed of roses, and all the chocolates you can eat. But on the left, the nasty vacuum cleaner of defeat sucks you down into Terrible Failure.

Who takes care of that vacuum cleaner? Somebody had to plug it into the wall. Somebody changes its vacuum cleaner bags. Somebody pointed it in your general direction. But who? Perhaps it was you. Sure you may have critics, detractors, and generally bad people who want to see you fail, but you plugged the vacuum in yourself if you let them get to you.

I always feel as if I'm on the verge of one of these two things: great Success or great Nothingness. In other words, there's the tiniest possibility that I'll make something really worthwhile of my life, but that bit of hope is eclipsed by the idea that I will try and try to accomplish something important only to end up old and frustrated instead. It's usually all I can do not to give up and throw myself down the left side of the mountain, where I'd be, lazy and anonymous in my flannel pajamas and watching *Seinfeld* reruns every day after my 8-to-5 day job. That hasn't happened . . . yet.

Happily, there's a little secret about the right side of the mountain: success begets success. It's one of the greatest motivators. Let's say you go out and buy a metal detector, make a few passes over an interesting patch of ground, and find an old Masonic trinket. The excitement of your find gives you the energy and impetus to continue looking for treasure. On the other hand, what if you spend an hour or more sweeping over the ground with nothing to show for it? Your arm starts to ache from the weight of the metal detector. You start to think this was a dumb idea, that it was a goofy waste of money—not to mention your time. Eventually you may consign the device—along with dreams of exciting finds—to the garage forevermore. Just as success begets success, failure, unfortunately, begets failure.

THE DIFFERENCE BETWEEN WHAT IS AND WHAT COULD BE

My old friend Steve impaled himself on the Precipice of Success. He was so afraid of failure and so afraid of success that he got stuck right at the top.

After he graduated from college, he moved back in with his parents. He spent all of his time writing and recording songs which can't be categorized or easily described. Simply put, they were wonderful. And there were hundreds of them. His songs were whimsical gifts that most people will never get to hear. Here's why:

He used to tell me that you have to know when to give up. He said dreamers are people who will never be happy, and he was sure he'd never be "successful." I'm not sure what his definition of success was, but I have a hunch it was pretty narrow and unrealistic. It really doesn't matter what "success" must have meant for him since he never actively marketed himself or his music. Although I'm sure he probably would've enjoyed a modest career as a musician, he was unwilling to risk being unhappy doing what he thought he wanted to do.

While I was working on *The Lost Soul Companion,* he sold his instruments and his recording equipment. He bought a suit, took the LSAT, and now plans to enroll in law school. Now we can be certain he won't fail as a musician. And the world gets another lawyer.

THE TRUTH ABOUT "SUCCESS"

The difference between what is and what could be is almost entirely up to you. It may not seem like it, but you have a lot of control over your own success or failure.

The only difference between an "author" and an aspiring writer is that someone, somewhere, thought that the author's work was worth being published. But having your work validated in the "real world" doesn't really mean that you've arrived, that you're talented, or worthy of great acclaim. Contrary to popular belief, it certainly isn't a reflection of your abilities as a writer, artist, musician, filmmaker . . . your talent with whatever it is that you live to do.

A while back, I heard that some clever people decided to take John Steinbeck's novel *The Grapes of Wrath* and turn it into an anonymous-looking manuscript, changing only the author's name and the book's title. They then sent the manuscript out to a bunch of agents and publishers across the country to see what would happen. It was rejected across the board. As the story goes, this great classic wasn't recognized by literary agents and editors as *The Grapes of Wrath*! Urban legend or not, the tale seems plausible, and that in itself says quite a lot about the publishing industry. Timing, luck, and salability are everything.

Without an audience or feedback from other people, a lot of creative people feel they haven't yet really "arrived." And many don't have the umph to finish what they've started all on their own. We all require some amount of external motivation, but be prepared. You won't always get what you need.

PROCRASTINATION AND GETTING BACK ON THE HORSE

Sometimes when I sit down to write I just flake out. I fall into some kind of trance and start pulling at my hangnails until I am bleeding everywhere. Then, of course, I have to push my chair back, stand up, walk to the bathroom, turn on the light, open the medicine cabinet, select the perfect Band-Aid, unwrap said Band-Aid and affix it to the wounded area. Then I glance up, notice a pimple on my chin or next to my eyebrow. It must be dealt with now. It cannot wait. I work at it with unparalleled concentration, coaxing the rewarding goo out of its reddened nest only to be left with a much more noticeable bruisy splotch in its place.

If only I could focus such attention on my writing!

But after the pimple I just feel dirty. Must shower. I'll get back to my writing later. Another time. Really soon though. (Honestly I have no idea how I got through college.) What's so hard about writing? I don't know, but if it were easy then everyone would be publishing books and it would no longer seem so special to me. The oddest part? Once you do get back on the horse, it can be great. Your horse can be galloping along sporting an enormous erection and, you imagine, a barely perceptible smile on his horsy face.

But mostly there are those nights when I end up with Band-Aids on every single finger and my horse has gone to sleep. Once when I worked as a temp at a photography studio, one of the other employees asked me why I had Band-Aids on nearly every finger. I lied. I told her I was an artist and I really got into my work. Maybe that's not such an exaggeration. It's true in a way.

As it turned out, she and her boyfriend were about to open an art gallery. They saw my work and offered me my own show. It was the start of something good. I think this is the only instance in my life when my procrastination coupled with dishonesty and a dash of obsessive-compulsive behavior had positive effects.

Nothing good has come of any of the other times I neglected my work so I'm trying to stop procrastinating so much. And I'm not the only one. My friend Paul, too, tries to be a writer, but he has lapses. Like the time he sat down at his desk to revise a draft of his latest novel. His chair squeaked a bit as he shifted his weight. He got his tools out, dismantled his chair, inspected it carefully, then put it all back together. This strenuous exercise exhausted him. A light nap was required. Poor thing.

Paul's MOST ridiculous procrastinations

If you procrastinate a lot, please don't feel too bad. Instead of writing, Paul spends an inordinate amount of time soaking in his bathtub where, he says, he gets some of his best ideas. The only problem is he can't jot them down in such a way as to be able to decipher them later. He thought he solved the problem when he bought a waxed pencil and started to write on the glass cutting board from his kitchen. It seemed to work quite well so he ran a bath, prepared his customary bowl of grapes, and climbed in. He told me he came up with some fantastic ideas, but, once the cutting board got wet, they slid right off into his bath.

Once he stood on top of his swivel office chair to determine if he could spin himself around only by flapping his arms. It worked.

Sometimes he paces his little room lecturing on the subject of African development to an imaginary audience. He even taught himself how to read hieroglyphics.

I, too, am a shameless procrastinator. While I can't begin to explain Paul's bizarre behavior, I have come to understand my own. There were a few sections of this book which I found myself putting off again and again until they were all that were left to do. Once I began to tackle them, I realized that I had been putting them off with good reason. Sometimes I procrastinated because writing the sections was going to be emotionally difficult for me, and part of my brain knew this and tried to hide that fact from the rest of me. Mine is a kind, well-meaning brain. When there are difficult emotions to face, it just wants to shut down. That can be problematic for my writing—especially since my best work leaves me naked for everyone to see.

I wasted months halfheartedly searching for information on phatic communication in order to write a clever and perfect introduction to this book. Granted, I didn't ask anyone else for help. I could've probably just called around and pestered people in the outside world until I found the information I required. Now I believe I was afraid I would find what I was looking for! Unless I found exactly what I thought I needed, I wouldn't really have to get started on the writing itself. And if I didn't get started on the writing, then I couldn't finish *The Lost Soul Companion* anytime soon, and then no one would be able to pick it up, read it, and, naturally, think it was really stupid.

Fear has a way of keeping us from doing what it is we want to do. A little procrastination now and then is one thing, but if you consistently neglect what's supposed to be your life's work—your painting, your fiction, your music, your acting, your anything—then something just isn't quite right. It may be time to ask yourself some hard questions.

How badly do I want this? What exactly am I trying to do? What is my goal again? Can I really do this? Will it be PERFECT? what if i fail?

THE CHOPSTICK PLAN

Paul doesn't procrastinate nearly so much since he implemented his chopstick plan. I have the smiley/frowny/straight-line face plan, but first, Paul's.

He got a pickle jar and filled it with fifteen chopsticks—exactly the number of chapters he had left to revise. Every time he finished one of his chapters, he removed a chopstick from the jar. It became a concrete reminder of his task.

Similarly, I have a dry-erase board on which I sketch a giant calendar. At the end of every day, I draw a face in the date square. A smiley face means I did lots of good writing that day. A face with a straight-line mouth means I did some research or prep work but no actual writing. A frowny face means I blew everything off completely. A frowny face with Xs over the eyes means I had terrible cramps and was incapacitated. You wouldn't think so, but a whole line of frowns in a row can be rather motivating.

GETTING MOTIVATED . . . BE AFRAID

Fear is a terrific motivator. So is the prospect of public humiliation. The two are closely related, and both can dramatically increase your productivity.

First the general kind of fear. I once rented a room in a beautiful Victorian house that was much more than I could reasonably afford. I knew that I didn't make enough money at my regular job to cover all of my expenses, so I'd have to compensate by creating and selling lots of artwork—something I had been meaning to do anyway.

It was sink or swim, and, somehow, I swam. Necessity dictated that I work my butt off. I had two large exhibits that year instead of just one. And I had work on consignment in shops. I produced some fantastic work because if I didn't, I'd be out on the street.

When we take risks and put all of our energy into something, the universe will reward us—sooner or later.

My friend Benjamin is best motivated by the prospect of public humiliation. He and his brother used to convince nightclubs to give them stand-up comedy gigs—even though they actually had nothing in particular to perform. The night before they were to go onstage, they would lock themselves in a room and write well into the morning. Sleep-deprived and terrified, they came up with some very successful bits.

Fear and apprehension can be the Lost Soul's friends.

KNOWING WHEN TO GIVE UP

Some people think there's a time and a place to give up on their dreams, but I don't agree. I've discovered that there's always a time and a place to reevaluate your goals— and reevaluating your goals is a completely different animal from the give-up-altogether animal.

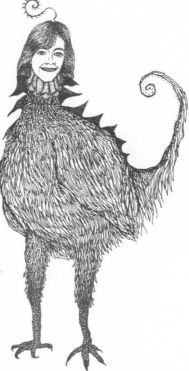

Experience necessitates this kind of revision. Consider the millions of girls growing up in the 1970s, dreaming of marrying Shaun Cassidy. As they got older—and wiser— I'll bet most of them decided they didn't want to marry a former teen heartthrob.

Decide whether or not your goals—factoring in a lot of hard work and some luck, too—are attainable. And decide if you still want to attain them at all.

There's nothing wrong with changing your expectations. And you can even take a rest from what you're trying to accomplish once in a while. If you think your only options are giving up your dreams completely or single-handedly accomplishing everything you ever wanted to on the very first try, then you're wrong, baby, wrong. What about the middle-of-the-road approach? After all, there isn't just one middle road. There are millions of avenues to take. When is it time to give up? Never. When is it time to readjust things? Anytime you feel the need.

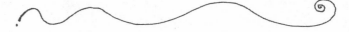

KENNY THE REDHEADED BASS PLAYER ON "MAKING IT BIG"

My old friend Kenny has been in eleven different bands. (Sometimes three or four at once!) He would never say that he "made it big" as a musician, but he sure has gotten close. There would've been no stopping him if it weren't for the fact that he looked "making it big" in the face and then changed his mind. His expertise on bass guitar enabled him to tour parts of Europe with the band Velo Deluxe, but after a while Kenny was ready to come home, maybe go back to school, and play for smaller audiences at local clubs.

When I asked him why he came back he explained that touring was very hard—"grueling" was his word. He was often disoriented because he and the rest of the band drove five or six hours a day, stopping just long enough to perform, crash in a hotel around 5 A.M., check out by 11 A.M., and then do it all over the next day. He got sick of playing the same songs over and over, but when you're on tour, that's what it takes. In Kenny's case, that old saying "Be careful what you wish for because you just might get it" really applies. The thrill of the chase is what motivated him. The minute he got what he wanted, it all started looking pretty dull.

If you want to "make it big" in the music business,

you'd better be sturdy. If huge commercial success is important to you, then you have to be willing to deal with what Kenny calls "some gross and annoying levels" of the industry. You must be prepared to market yourself, deal with managers, tour constantly, and possibly be disappointed along the way. He cheerily remarked, "Most people fail. Everyone wants to think, 'Well, I'm not the failure. If I have a positive attitude something will happen . . .' No. Some of the best bands in the world don't get anywhere."

Kenny says about 90 percent of the greatest songwriters in the world have never been heard. They freaked out somewhere in the initial stages of making it big. The most talented songwriter he knows is a guy named Marty. Marty is a carpenter who plays his guitar on street corners for bottles of wine; Marty says he's relatively happy, and that's good enough for him.

THE FLEXIBLE AND OPEN-MINDED MICHAEL TEAGUE

Michael Teague told me he lives in the same building with a Peeping Tom, and he has to share his bathroom with a bulimic. He's also one of the best artists I know. If I could give him a house of his own, I would.

Working part-time hours in order to have time for painting and drawing, he's among the underemployed and it's starting to wear on him.

He made the comic that follows, "Second Chance," featuring the Glitter Glue Fairy, just for *The Lost Soul Companion* project. He's extremely generous and very talented, and, everyone reading this, mark my words: Michael Teague is going places!

For the most part, he's a comix artist, but he didn't start out that way. He had a friend who was writing a novel, and the two got into the habit of visiting The Runcible Spoon, a local coffee shop.

"My friend wanted me to come to the Spoon with him," Michael explained, "because he wanted companionship while he was working on his novel. When I first started hanging out there, I would bring a notebook and maybe scribble some really rough comic or something like that.

"I really wasn't even intending to think of myself as a comix artist. I was still thinking of myself as a painter because I had just gotten my MFA and spent $12,000 so I had better be a painter.

"The thing is I started drawing and every day I would come in and draw something else and before you know it I was making full-length comix. Around that time I remember my friend went back to California for a year and I

SECOND CHANCE

featuring the **Glitter Glue Fairy** *by m. l. teague 1999*

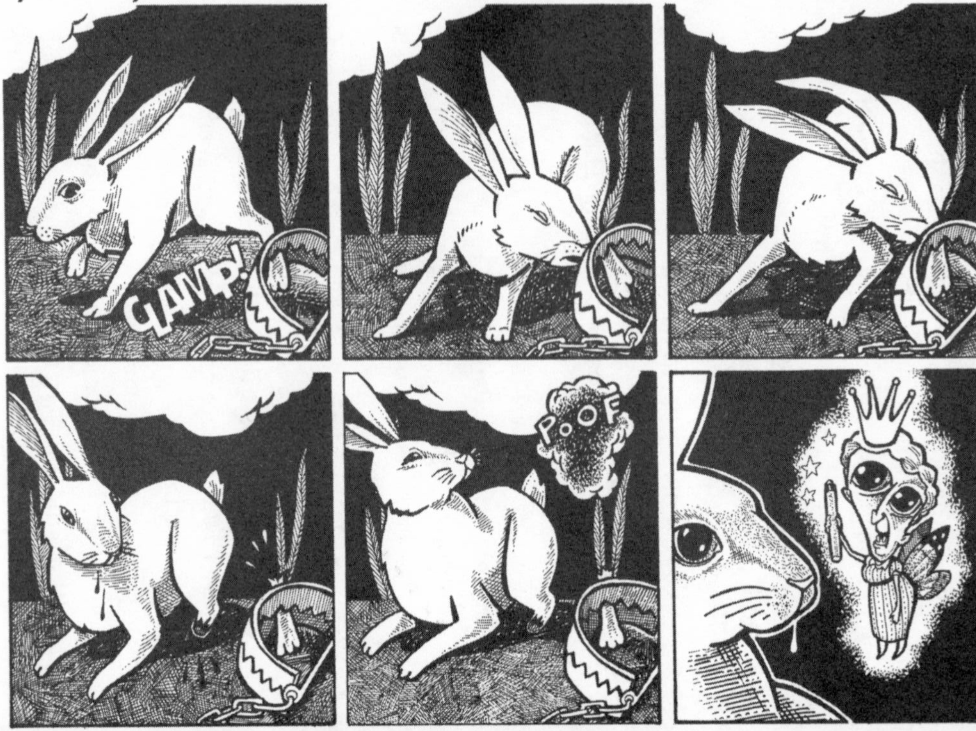

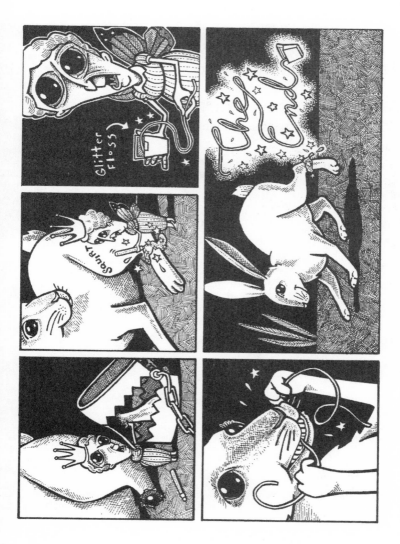

kept going to the Spoon and making comix. I had created forty or fifty pages of one-page comix drawn in ballpoint pen. I dedicated that first book to him.

"During the course of making that first book—without really being aware of it—I created the entire skeleton of what would be the foundation for my present work. I touched on everything in terms of plot, my writing style, hinting at my future drawing style . . . things of that nature."

I like the fact that Michael stumbled upon this passion by accident. Even though he is supposed to be a painter* (because he spent lots of money to study to be one), he let himself try something new. And even though it hasn't paid off in the same ways that his painting has— at least not yet—he still indulges in his comix habit. That is why I call him the flexible and open-minded Michael Teague.

---

* *Michael told me he would like to be a footnote in an art history book someday. For now he is a footnote in* The Lost Soul Companion. *He still paints. He has had gallery shows in Chicago, New York, and Los Angeles, and his paintings have sold for thousands of dollars. Still, I think he likes making comix more than painting.*

THICK SKIN AND BAD PRESS

I wrote a letter to Rush Limbaugh, but he didn't write me back. I wanted to know how he got such thick skin—how it is that he's able to handle criticism so well. Maybe he didn't want me to have the secret. Or maybe my letter got wedged inside the postbox in such a way as to remain undiscovered all this time. Anyway, I, like many Lost Souls, am overly sensitive to every kind of criticism.

I bristle at the constructive kind, and the especially nasty type—that which is not at all constructive—can ruin me for weeks. The truth is, I'm one of the worst people to offer any advice on it. However, for you, I'll try.

Constructive criticism isn't so hard to handle if I think of it as a rare gift from some well-meaning person. In a way, that's what it is. If I get mixed reviews in the press, for example (and I have . . .), I'm best served by taking away valid suggestions for improving my art and by feeling flattered that the reviewer thought enough of my work to mention it at all.

As for the really scathing, unconstructive kind of criticism, I hide under my bed for a couple of days. When I decide to come out it is usually because I have carefully considered my critic's motivation.

Maybe he has a personal problem that I couldn't even begin to understand. Maybe he secretly wants to paint clown portraits but can't. Some critics are just mean-spirited. Don't give them or their caustic criticism any power. Pity them and move on.

THE WHITE STATUE-MAN

I saw the white statue-man downtown on Pacific Mall Avenue in Santa Cruz, California. He was wearing long, white elbow gloves, a white hood, and a long, white robe. His face was painted white—even his lips and eyelashes—and he must've been standing up on something under the robe because he looked really, really tall. He stood perfectly still. There was a ceramic bowl on a small platform at his feet to collect money, and anytime someone put money in the bowl, he briefly came to life. I was with my ex-boyfriend and his kids at the time. When the kids saw the statue-man come to life they asked us if he was real or a machine. That's how good he was! He would open his eyes and move his head and arms very gracefully in a gesture of thanks to anyone who had just dropped money into his bowl. It was absolutely mesmerizing. Then he would go back to being completely still, eyes shut, head bowed, hands together. He looked really peaceful and kind. There was a huge crowd admiring him. One after another people came to bring him money . . . and he would wake up again. His performance was one of the neatest things I have ever seen. His ability to draw and captivate a crowd was amazing. There must have been thirty or forty people standing around, quietly admiring him. His concentration was perfect.

He must have had things pretty well together because he never even cracked a smile when he was "off" and one lady in the crowd began to heckle him. She had a meaty face topped with dark, curly hair, and the minute she began to speak, I had the feeling that no one in the crowd liked her one bit. I certainly didn't. Clearly, she was trying to get the statue-man to mess up. I think she was a little crazy. She started singing this mocking little song—quietly at first then louder and louder—swaying her hips and scrunching up her face. I can still hear her terrible singing in my head. The song went something like this: "Gotta earn some money in Santa Cruz . . . Lookin' pretty pale in Santa Cruz . . . How ya gonna live in Santa Cruz? . . . Got nowhere to go in Santa Cruz . . ." and so on.

My cynical side wonders if she was planted in the audience to elicit sympathy for the statue-man because the crowd began dropping more coins—and even large bills—into his collection bowl at an incredible rate after she began her heckling. (Statue-man, if you get a copy of this book, won't you please write and tell me if she was part of your act? And then will you have dinner with me?) It was the crowd's way of showing support for the creative, gentle, and beautifully mute soul who stood before us. But with each clink of coins in the bowl, her singing sounded louder, more grating than before. Folks in the crowd started yelling at the woman to shut up and go away, but she wouldn't budge. I didn't stay to find out what happened. By now I'm sure the statue-man has gone home. As for the heckler, for all I know she is still standing on Pacific Mall Avenue, hips swaying, under a cloud of her own making.

Whenever someone tries to hurt me or belittle my creative efforts for their own gain, all I have to do is think of the white statue-man's grace and composure on that day and I feel calmer, more in control of my situation.

3.

Creative Coping

PANHANDLERS: GIVING
UNDEREMPLOYMENT A BAD NAME

One thing I really despised about Santa Cruz was the panhandling. Every few blocks on Pacific Mall Avenue there were people—often very young and seemingly able-bodied—with their hands outstretched, holding rough cardboard signs that read, "No food. No money. No place to go. Please help. God bless."

These people always asked me for money because I was pounding the pavement in my best outfit, little portfolio in hand, looking desperately for work. They must've thought I had something to give, but honestly I wasn't much better off than any of them. I felt guilty for not giving them the last of my money, and I resented them, too, for having put me in that awkward position to begin with.

I might have given them the change in my pocket if they had at least attempted to make some contribution to the community. But they didn't strum guitars or read poems or draw beautiful pictures with chalk on the sidewalk in exchange for tips.

Alexander the Great conquered most of the known world before he turned thirty-three. What did these people ever do? Where are their inner resources?

I couldn't figure out exactly why I resented them so much, but now I know. They are giving underemployment a bad name.

I have been "underemployed" more often than not, choosing self-employment and temp work over a more traditional—and stable—existence. And even now that I work a forty-hour-a-week, "straight" job, I still feel underemployed because I have passed over opportunities for higher

a word about street performers...

Santa Cruz did have lots of great street performers, and I supported them as much as I could because I think they enrich communities in many intangible ways.

75

pay and advancement in exchange for less responsibility (read: fewer headaches!) and more flexible hours (management can't always duck out early on a Friday afternoon . . .). As a result of my choices, I am officially below the poverty line. Nonetheless, I live well, and you won't find me panhandling on the street.

QUIT YOUR DAY JOB?
BILL ROBERTSON AND DAZEY THE COW

My friend Bill is an electrical engineer, an artist, and a musician. He never limits himself. He loves to do a little of this and a little of that. Some people are really disturbed by his work, but I'm delighted by it.

Not long after I met him he showed me a short video he made called "The Puppet Show." You may have seen it on a compilation video called *N D 11*. He casually refers to it as his roadkill video. A weird old song started the whole thing. It was a twelfth-century French piece ironically called "The Frog Song." It's an odd woodwind arrangement of only four grating notes. It inspired Bill to create his video, which is ghastly, patently offensive, and also quite charming.

In case you missed "The Puppet Show," imagine an

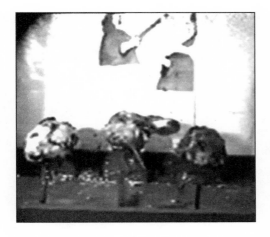 elaborate Punch and Judy–type puppet stage complete with blood-spattered curtains. The curtains part, revealing four animals' disembodied heads impaled on sticks. (Not to worry, the animals were roadkill and, according to Bill, "long since dead when we scraped them up for auditions.") The stars were, from left to right, an opossum, a rabbit, a groundhog, and a squirrel. Each head corresponded with one of the four notes of "The Frog Song." (The opossum represented the lowest note because he had the biggest head and so on.) Each time they heard their animal's corresponding note, the four "animal head manipulators" underneath the puppet stage would thrust their animal heads up through the bottom of the stage basin, which, by the way, was filled with chocolate pudding. I think you have to see "The Puppet Show" to really appreciate it. It's macabre and cute at the same time. I never thought that was possible.

After his work with the roadkill was done, Bill gave them a proper burial. (You see, he is a sensitive and kind man.)

The roadkill video led Bill to his best work ever: Dazey the cow. Bill explained, "I took the roadkill video I made into work and showed it to some people in the conference room and one guy said, 'Well, I know where there is a complete cow skeleton at the farmer's place who lives right next to me.' He drew me a map and I went out there and there was this complete cow skeleton." Our conversation went like this:

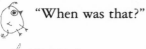 "When was that?"

"1991."

"And the farmer let you have it?"

"The farmer never knew about it. His neighbor—my friend—took care of it for me. I got it back here and I was just going to put it together and leave it in the living room, and then as I was starting to process all the bones and stuff I figured I would mechanize it—make it mobile rather than just sitting around. That way it's kind of nice that your art can move around rather than just hang on a wall or sit there and be stared at.

"The bones were in pretty good shape. They

had been sitting out for so long that animals had come along and eaten all the meat off of them so that there was hardly anything left . . . Part of the spinal column was still connected together with nasty connecting tissue and gristle and all that stuff so I had to hammer and chisel it apart. Basically all the meat and everything was completely gone. All the hair was gone so it was pretty nice. I just soaked it in bleach water for forty-eight hours in a big vat of water with several gallons of bleach in it and then had to scrub on it and take a grinding wheel and a drill and grind off all of the little connecting tissue things."

 "How long did that take?"

 "Processing the bones took several weeks. Then I just started putting them together. I put the spinal column together first and hung it from the ceiling and started attaching legs and stuff."

 "Why did you do it?"

 "It's art. It just felt like I needed to. It was there. It was an evolution of what I've been working with. Doing roadkill stuff—in a nice, tasteful way, of course—and then just going into bone art. I've always been intrigued by primitive art—especially when bones are involved. So I kind of wanted to do the thing to where it's a blend between technology and real primitive art."

 "Have you ever tried to sell your art?"

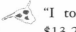 "I took Dazey out once with a price tag of $13,273. I would have sold her for $13,273."

 "You wouldn't have missed her?"

 "Sure I would've missed her, but I would've sold her."

 "How did you arrive at that number?"

 "I figured I had $273 in parts and the $13,000 is labor."

Dazey is still for sale. I think she's a bargain.

From preparing and assembling the bones to articulating and motorizing Dazey's skeleton, Bill spent about fourteen months on the project. "When I was working on Dazey," Bill told me, "I had a live-in girlfriend, I was in one regular full-time band and one part-time band, and

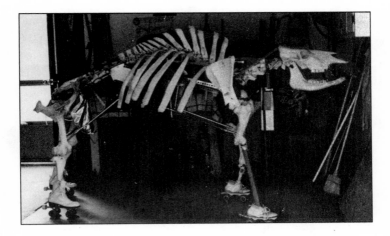

then working forty hours a week, but I would come home from work and I would change clothes and head straight out to the garage and work and I'd do that every day . . . I was into the project too much to be tired. I get obsessed when I'm really into something. I forget to eat because I get busy. You get hungry for a moment but then it passes really quickly because you're thinking about [your work]."

His next project is going to be fantastic, but he made me promise to keep it a secret. I think he wants us to be surprised.

I asked him if he regrets getting his engineering degree and going to a "real job" every day and he said no, you have to eat; you have to buy supplies. "That's why I got a straight job," he explained, "so that I could pay for stuff and then I could play whatever music I wanted to and didn't have to struggle and play crap I hated just to be able to eat and be a professional musician."

So how do you know when to quit your day job—or when to get a day job? I tend to be in favor of having a "real job" because, in my case, I really need the health insurance—without which I would be spending about $90 a month on my antidepressant medication instead of just $12—and some amount of structure in my day. The steady, albeit small, paycheck is nice too. Plus I must interact with other people, bathe, and change my clothes regularly. All good aspects to the day job.

Of course living in the "real world" with a "real job" can suck too. Some days I barely have the energy to drive myself home—let alone work on any of my own creative projects. I long for great blocks of free time, and, once you factor in doing the laundry, paying the bills, cooking, and grocery shopping, weekends don't really count.

There are always good reasons to have a day job, and there are great reasons to quit your day job, but why don't more people consider simply changing their day jobs? If you are an artist working as, say, a telemarketer and you hate it (imagine that!), why not offer private art lessons instead? Or teach at your local community arts center, or, perhaps, be an artsy activities director at a retirement home? You might find this work more rewarding than selling sets of encyclopedias over the telephone, and it could pay off in a number of ways. Since you might enjoy your new line of work more, you'd be more relaxed and ready to take on your own projects when you get home. Also, your students and others in the community would begin to recognize your talents and learn more about your work and your artistic aesthetic. I bet those topics never would've come up at your old job.

So if you're miserable at work, get out. Life's too short for that. But if you're only slightly miserable at work—and you're still able to do a little of this and that at the end of the day—that's not half bad.

"MODELING WHILE MOVING"

Some Lost Souls find themselves far away from home, waiting and hoping to be discovered as actors. (Or, for that matter, waiting and hoping to become famous artists, writers, and so on . . .) Is this you? Or a Lost Soul you know? I had the opportunity to pick a working actor's brain one afternoon, so maybe the following will help.

His name is Mark, and he told me that there are a couple different kinds of often out-of-work actors.

According to him, the first kind even has a name. He explained, "So many guys say, 'Oh, I'd like to do theater and film, but I really don't want to do TV.' No one ever thinks about wanting to do commercials or anything like that. That kind of thinking tends to create the 'Theater Snob' with these unreal expectations."

The other kind of actor comes to L.A. or New York expecting to be a movie star even though he lacks the proper training or experience. He continued, "Neither of those are prepared to look at all the different aspects of making money in acting. Not that we aspire to be commercial actors—doing voice-overs or CD-ROM or whatever—but that's the whole change of thought that I had. I'd rather do that kind of acting to feed myself while I'm trying to do film or great theater acting because I don't think one medium is superior to the other. I'd rather do good TV than bad theater. People say they don't want to do TV but then they're doing crappy independent films that are terribly written. Just because it's an independent film doesn't make it good." Of course there are good indies out there, but what if you don't get the perfect part? How can you get by until your inevitable big break?

There are viable alternatives to waiting tables, and you don't have to sell yourself on the streets either. Just accept that you have to start small. You may even have to do some (gasp!) commercial work. The best advice I've come across seems oversimplified, but it makes a lot of sense. You want to be an actor? You'll have to acquire experience—even if you don't think it really counts.

Consider the "industrial films"—the kind that aren't for public broadcast. Companies produce them to train and educate their employees. They're essential and ubiquitous. There are the accident safety videos, inventory procedure films, and, of course, sexual harassment programs, to name a few. (Mark performed this line expertly: "Hey, Jack, I don't know if Elaine appreciates your advances . . .") He has made $500 a night doing these kinds of projects.

He has done television commercials, too. "Commercials are a whole different thing," he said. "Even if you do a good commercial, it's not really acting that I'd call it. It's modeling while moving . . ." Like it or not, it pays the bills. Not only do you get paid for your time on the set, you also can make residuals every time the commercial airs.

And remember that you really can be someone in your own backyard. Would-be actors don't have to move to L.A. or New York to get acting jobs. It seems that every city, to some extent, makes local radio and television commercials. It may not be glamorous, but there is work to be had if you really want it. Mark recommends sending your resume and professional headshot to local talent agents or, if there are none, then directly to advertising agencies, or even to potential clients themselves. He has also contacted local television stations directly, and he has gotten auditions as a result.

Radio voice-overs can also be a good source of income.

To get radio voice-over work, you'll need a good demo tape. You can invest in professional studio time or borrow a friend's good sound equipment. If you lack examples of your radio ability, listen to some existing spots, then improve on them to use for your demo. Send your tapes off to area ad agencies along with your resume and contact information.

Finally, if you really want to move away from home to pursue your acting career, you may not have to move thousands of miles to do it. If you live in or near a city that has regional theater, you're set. Just think, much of your competition is busy scrambling for parts in one of two cities bursting with out-of-work actors.

I have noticed that people can be very weird about money. So if you are thinking, "Where does she get off trying to tell me how to spend my money," skip this part. Maybe it's not for you.

CREATIVITY AND POVERTY

For most Lost Souls who choose some kind of career in the arts, the best we can hope for is having just enough money to get by. That's not to say that the life of an artist, musician, writer, actor, or whatever you are can't be a rich one. It can . . . just maybe not in the traditional sense.

There are some tricks to living comfortably on very little income. I am able to save exactly half of my monthly earnings because:

I never let my rent exceed one week's pay (or at least not by much . . .). Since I make about $300 a week after taxes, I looked and looked for a place in that range. I settled for a $325-a-month hole-in-the-wall. It was a "cute studio apartment" next door to a detox center. There were hornets living in one of the walls.

But, after we got the bugs worked out, it wasn't so bad.

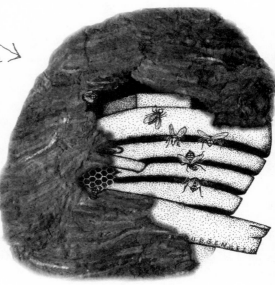

I saw the nest after the maintenance man finally took the plywood siding off of one side of the house. The hornets had made their own version of the Guggenheim. It was impressive!

And the men at the detox center kept a close eye on my place. One guy was an ex-mechanic who sometimes helped me with my car problems.

The sacrifices I make now enable me to keep doing what I want to do—my art and writing on my time. And although I could probably afford a nicer place, I'm willing to delay my gratification, save my money, and buy a small house of my own someday.

2 I pay my credit card bill off in full every month. The credit card companies call people like me "deadbeats." My card has no annual fee, and, because I never go the minimum payment route, the credit card people don't even make interest off me. (I almost feel sorry for them . . . almost.)

I usually pay for necessities such as groceries and gas with my card because I like getting the itemized statement at the end of the month. It makes keeping track of my spending habits really easy—and I don't have to carry around lots of cash or pay with checks all the time. (Not to mention the fact that I am establishing a good credit rating for later.)

I know this may sound oversimplified, but the trick is not spending more money than you know you can earn. I've made a reasonable budget for myself, and I stick to it.

For Lost Souls with enough discipline, a credit card can provide a monthly, interest-free loan.

 I barter whenever possible. I have traded my artwork for rent, bicycles, and one whole summer of fresh vegetables. And bartering really saved my skin in Santa Cruz. When I needed a place to stay, the manager of Caffe Pergolessi let me stay at his house in exchange for doing the dishes and keeping the place tidy. Thank you! Thank you!

 I don't go to the mall. A lot of people go shopping just for fun. When I do that, I risk feeling deprived. I see a CD I'd really like to have or a little dress that I think I can't live without. It must be all of the lavender air freshener they pump into those places that makes me want to part with so much of my money so quickly. Or maybe it's the artful color scheme or the fact that a store has decorated their interior with a distressed chain-link fence. I love it. I want it all. And so I stay home.

When I really do start to feel deprived, I enter contests to win stuff off the radio. All the different stations are always having contests of some kind. I have won CDs, restaurant gift certificates, and concert tickets that way. Those extravagances are even better when they are free.

I try to anticipate my needs and plan ahead. One of my biggest expenses used to be matting and framing my artwork. Getting ready for an exhibit or art fair really stretched my financial resources to their limit. I solved the problem by doing everything backwards. Now, instead of having custom frames built to fit my artwork, I buy used frames at garage sales and secondhand stores, and create the art to fit my frames.

Occasionally the frames I find are so extraordinary that they inspire entire artworks all by themselves. Sometimes my dad helps me refinish or resize them if they need a little extra attention to be glorious again.

Anticipating my needs in this way has saved me hundreds and hundreds of dollars. Also, I'm able to sell my framed originals at reasonable prices so that all kinds of people can afford to start their own art collections. I have sold my work to teachers, waitresses, college students, farmers, and even other artists. Knowing that they didn't have much in the way of expendable income made those sales even more gratifying.

 I am careful with myself. My parents have always reminded me not to do anything stupid. I still do plenty of stupid things, but these are a few I've been able to avoid:

• I don't smoke, and if I did, I'd say the cigarette companies should be paying me to use their abominable products and not the other way around.

• I rarely drink because alcohol and antidepressants really don't mix well. A little alcohol in moderation can be a very good thing, but I've seen too many people waste a lot of time and money on firewater. The same can be said of other recreational drugs.

• I don't have cable TV. It rates right up there with smoking. I think we should go live our lives instead of just watching imitation life on TV. (And we can all save thirty bucks a month or more while we're at it.)

The one really smart thing I always do: buy health insurance. It has often been a hardship for me—especially when I was entirely self-employed—but I would never want to go without at least very basic health insurance. You just never know when you'll need it, and if you don't have some kind of coverage, you could be paying off hospital bills for the rest of your life.

The corollary to buying health insurance is practicing preventive medicine, which has gotten me some breaks on my insurance premiums. Always wearing my seatbelt in cars counts in this category.

Getting plenty of sleep, eating relatively well (I don't really . . .), taking vitamins (sporadically . . .), and using

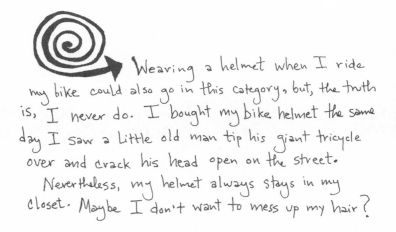 Wearing a helmet when I ride my bike could also go in this category, but, the truth is, I never do. I bought my bike helmet the same day I saw a little old man tip his giant tricycle over and crack his head open on the street.

Nevertheless, my helmet always stays in my closet. Maybe I don't want to mess up my hair?

echinacea (an herb which I believe strengthens the immune system) at the first signs of cold or flu (always!) are my old standbys. (I guess you could say there is always room for improvement.)

Strength in Numbers

One great way to get by is to start a collective. Find two or three other struggling souls in your community and pool your resources. Buy staples, paper goods, and other necessities in bulk, and then divvy them up accordingly.

Lost Souls and Food

I never have much food in my house. Many Lost Souls don't. I'm lucky to have a bag of dried-out onions, a jar of pickles, moldy cheese, and maybe curry powder. I don't have a lot of food because I don't budget a lot of money for it—and I don't have the time or inclination to go to the store regularly.

Even when I *have* had plenty of raw ingredients, I have sobbed uncontrollably at the thought of peeling a potato or boiling water for pasta. It all required more energy than I actually had. (Ironically, I lacked energy because I did not eat well enough.) Also, I generally prefer spending my time on my art or writing instead of mixing or frying or baking anything or washing dishes. Still, I've learned, we all have to eat sooner or later.

THE TOASTER OVEN
WAS MY SALVATION

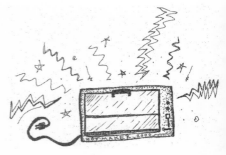

Toaster ovens are inexpensive and indispensable. Every Lost Soul needs one. I use mine every morning and nearly every night. Some toaster oven recipes for really hungry, really lazy Lost Souls:

VEGGIE REUBEN SANDWICH

you need: two slices of bread, Muenster or mozzarella cheese, one can of sauerkraut, and a bottle of Thousand Island dressing

Place part of the can of sauerkraut and a slice of cheese on bread, sprinkle with Thousand Island dressing, put other slice of bread on top. Toast in toaster oven until sandwich is hot and melty. You're done!

LITTLE FAKE PIZZAS

you need: English muffins (pita bread is good, too), spaghetti sauce, grated mozzarella cheese, and pepperoni

Spread spaghetti sauce over the English muffin. Sprinkle with cheese, finish with pepperoni (or some other topping if you prefer). Toast in toaster oven until pizza is hot and melty. You're done!

THE OBVIOUS TOASTED CHEESE SANDWICH

you need: two slices of bread, whatever cheese you like; optional: tomato, spinach, ham, or some other kind of meat, if that's what you eat

Place cheese on bread (if you have it, add tomato, spinach, ham, or whatever you think would be good on a toasted cheese sandwich), put other slice of bread on top. Toast in toaster oven until sandwich is hot and melty. You're done!

AND SOME NON–TOASTER-OVENY IDEAS

BREAKFAST FOR DINNER

Scramble some eggs or have a bowl of cereal. Anything is better than nothing!

HOMEMADE GRANOLA

you need: brown sugar, vegetable oil, honey, oatmeal, dry milk, cinnamon, and salt

When you have lots of extra energy, make a batch of granola in advance and be ready for your really uninspired cooking days. Mix ¾ cup brown sugar, ⅓ cup vegetable oil, and ⅓ cup honey in a saucepan and heat until the sugar is dissolved. Mix 3–4 cups of oats, ½ cup dry milk, ¾ teaspoon cinnamon, and a pinch of salt in a large cake pan. Pour the dissolved sugar over the dry ingredients and mix well. Bake at 375 degrees for 10 minutes. Let cool. Break up into little bits and store in a resealable Baggie or an airtight container. Lasts a fairly long time. You're done!

WHEN BOILING WATER ISN'T TOO MUCH TO ASK

THE VERY OBVIOUS MACARONI AND CHEESE

Macaroni and cheese is always an inexpensive, relatively quick option—especially if you have a microwave oven. And if you're really motivated, brown some ground beef (or textured vegetable protein), mix it in, and you're done! Not bad!

VALDA'S RAMEN NOODLE CONCOCTION

you need: ramen noodles (minus the nasty flavor packet that comes with them), frozen peas, curry powder, pepper, and one or two eggs

Boil a little bit of water; break the ramen noodles into little pieces and drop in. Stir eggs as you would for scrambled eggs and, when noodles are half done, drizzle eggs into the ramen noodles and stir. Add the frozen peas near the end—they don't need to cook long—just long enough to thaw out. Add curry powder and pepper to taste. Stir. You're done!

BLENDER FOOD

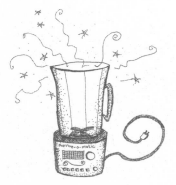

According to my friend Benjamin, if you have powdered milk and a blender, you can survive for a very long time. He says blender food is "expeditious with no tedious chewing." For Benjamin, blending carefully selected ingredients is an art form. For tired, hungry Lost Souls, it can be a lifesaving convenience.

THE BASIC SMOOTHIE

you need: eight ounces of water, 6 to 8 big ice cubes, ½ to 1 cup powdered milk, and ⅛ to ¼ cup raw oats and/or fresh tofu for texture and vitamins (optional)

Blend all that together for the basic smoothie base and then add your flavoring ingredients—chocolate, vanilla, coconut, peanut butter, bananas, mangoes, strawberries, peaches, carrots, etc.

The banana smoothie is especially economical because really old bananas work best. You can usually buy them for ten cents a pound, peel them, and store them in your freezer until it's smoothie time.

By the way, if regular milk doesn't agree with you, substitute rice, soy, or coconut milk.

The only problematic part about blender food is that it doesn't store well. Don't bother to make more than you will consume in one sitting. If you put your blender concoction in the fridge for later, it will stratify unpleasantly.

ONE MORE SNACKY THING . . .

Did you know that you can pop loose popcorn in your microwave in a plain paper bag? It's true. Just pour in enough popcorn to barely cover the bottom of the bag, fold about an inch of the top of the bag over, place the bag on its side, and nuke it one to three minutes (depending on your microwave . . .). Be sure to watch it the whole time. I left mine unattended for a bit too long. It took days to get the smell of burnt popcorn out of my hair—not to mention my cockatoo!

The nice thing about making popcorn this way is you get just plain popcorn without all the butter, salt, and artificial colors and flavors that often come with commercially prepared microwave popcorn, and you can add whatever you like yourself. People in Scotland put sugar on their popcorn—my Scottish friends thought the fact that we put salt on ours was strange. Anyway, you get more control over the whole popcorn experience. In the immortal words of Martha Stewart, it's a good thing.

LIVING THE RICH LIFE

In her excellent book called *Inspiration Sandwich* (read it!), SARK, a San Francisco-based artist, notes that "many people who have lots of money never feel rich." She continues, "Feeling rich is born of simple things: good health, comfort, freedom and laughter along with being well loved. Money is important but incidental. Remember this affirmation: you are welcome everywhere."

If you develop the right attitude you really are welcome everywhere. Although SARK is wildly successful (and probably fairly well off by now), she has not always had such sure economic footing. Nevertheless, she managed to live well. For instance, she has been visiting Paradise Island in the Bahamas for almost twenty years—even when she had next to nothing. She writes that she even slept on a chaise longue next to a swimming pool for two weeks because that's what she had access to at the time. I've always admired her ability to be comfortable anywhere, to adapt to her surroundings, and to court adventure.

I have applied SARK's ideas to my own life—albeit on a smaller scale. I know that "feeling rich" means different things to different people, and luxuries are relative. They can be dinners of scallops so tender that you feel like weeping, 300-thread-count sheets, fine cigars, a day at the spa . . . but warm, dry socks, air conditioning, and Heath bars are more my speed.

Although I love movies—especially first-runs in the theaters—I rarely go because I can't afford to. This may sound outlandish, but I've found a way around the problem of money. Employees of most movie theaters get some free passes fairly regularly. On certain occasions I've gotten in to see movies by offering ripe oranges, toy airplanes, and—my favorite—surprise packages of my creation in exchange for these guest passes. People love to help others—especially when it's easy for them. And, in this case, it is.

One evening I decided to try bartering with my fantastic Halloween Ball, a tantalizing mess of spider rings, wax lips, and chocolates inside a swirl of orange netting. I had waited in line for a little while and when it was my turn the young lady encased in the Plexiglas booth asked—for the umpteenth time that day, I'm sure—"which movie will it be?" I discreetly slid my ball of surprises through the little hole in the counter and asked if she would like to make a trade. (The moment I make this kind of offer to a movie ticket taker is always particularly magical. In fact, it's often better than the movie I came to see. Real life is better than the movies, but only if you really know how to live.) On her face, confusion turned to uncertainty, uncertainty to understanding, and, at last, magically, understanding turned into great delight. I like to think that she enjoyed a bright spot in what otherwise may have been a dull shift. She accepted my offer.

On a different occasion, I offered an enormous, fresh apple to a young man at the ticket booth; as it turned out, he told me he hadn't eaten all day and he was very happy to let me in.

Since then, I've made up a series of movie rules which I follow carefully. Anyone hoping to gain entry to a movie by wooing the ticket agent with pieces of fruit, pay close attention. 1. Use this kind of magic sparingly; you don't want to wear it out—nor do you want to wear out your welcome. 2. The exchange should be mutually pleasing and beneficial. You will only be truly welcome everywhere if you are a good person everywhere you go. 3. If the person behind the counter thinks you're crazy, you would be wise to pay them with real currency and quietly take a seat in the theater . . . but not before you give over the surprise you intended for them in the first place. It could make them feel a little better. This, in turn, will make you feel better too. If you ask me, that is real wealth.

TEMPLE GRANDIN AND THE SQUEEZE MACHINE

Being poor isn't the only challenge Lost Souls face. Some of us have trouble functioning in the outside world, but we can come up with our own good ways to cope. Temple Grandin did.

She was born with autism, and, while Lost Souls often feel unattached, few of us have experienced Temple's kind of isolation.

She says she feels like an anthropologist on Mars (she is featured in Oliver Sacks's excellent book of the same name, by the way) because she doesn't intuitively understand how other people think. Interpreting human feelings and motivations is nearly impossible for her. She negotiates day-to-day interactions by consulting a vast data bank in her head—not unlike Data, the robot in *Star Trek*. For Temple and other autistics like her, social convention often must be learned by rote. This is not to say that she is herself emotionless; on the contrary, she is capable of great compassion and even empathy. The creatures she understands best are animals—cattle, in particular.

Until the age of three, she was unable to speak, and it was thought that she would be institutionalized her whole life. Instead, she gradually learned to read. Temple developed a fascination with science, which eventually led to her professorship at Colorado State University. Now she travels and lectures both on animal behavior and autism. Temple Grandin is a role model for me because she has accomplished so much (too much to tell you about here!) and has lived so well . . . not to mention the fact that she is the inventor of the squeeze machine.

In her book *Thinking in Pictures,* she admits that, as a child, she hated to be hugged, but at the same time she craved the comfort such contact could offer. She writes, "When I was six, I would wrap myself up in blankets and get under sofa cushions, because the pressure was relaxing. I used to daydream for hours in elementary school about constructing a device that would apply pressure to my body . . . After visiting my aunt's ranch in Arizona, I got the idea of building such a device, patterned after the cattle squeeze chute I first saw there." One day Temple's aunt agreed to enclose her in the cattle squeeze chute to test its effects. Thirty minutes later, Temple emerged calmer and more relaxed. She explains, "This was the first time I ever really felt comfortable in my own skin." Not long after, she developed the first human squeeze machine.

Her prototype was made with plywood panels, but the latest design has padded side panels and a padded neck opening. Temple sent me this diagram:

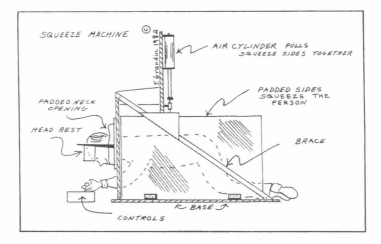

Despite pressure to get rid of her machine, Temple kept it in her room during college and continued to use it. The device helped ease her general anxiety and hypersensitivity to touch. The squeeze machine's therapeutic effects have even been documented, and, because the machine is now commercially available, many autistic people are benefiting from its use. (Anyone out there interested in buying their own squeeze machine, call the Therafin Corporation at 800-843-7234.)

I admire Temple Grandin's ingenuity, and I love the fact that she determined what it was that would improve the quality of her life—in this case, a hug machine, of all things!—and then she made her childhood dream a reality.

In *An Anthropologist on Mars,* she told Oliver Sacks, "I don't want my thoughts to die with me . . . I want to have done something . . . I'm not interested in power, or piles of money. I want to leave something behind. I want to make a positive contribution—know that my life has meaning . . ."

Because Temple was able to devise a coping mechanism of her own—and not be afraid to use it—she has been able to make a very positive contribution despite her personal challenges.

THE "WHAT COLOR IS YOUR MOTHER'S HAIR?" TEST OR HOW TO TELL IF SOMEONE IS LYING TO YOU

I don't always get along with others very well. I have trouble knowing when to trust people. For better or for worse, I've developed a few coping mechanisms of my own. They aren't quite as tangible as Temple Grandin's, and, admittedly, they're a little sneaky. But I have found that sometimes sneaky works best—especially when navigating the murky lagoon that is interpersonal relations . . .

By studying people's eye movements, I can usually tell when someone isn't being entirely honest with me. It goes something like this: If I'm talking with someone in person, I can ask them a simple, straightforward question like "What color is your mother's hair?" or "What was your first pet's name?" (or even a question you already know the answer to . . .), then watch which direction their eyes go in that instant in which they briefly search for the answer. Usually people look up and to the left or the right for half a second or so just before they say, "Blonde" or "Foofer."

Obviously, you don't want to tell them why you asked. I just work my question into the conversation naturally. Assuming they aren't likely to lie about the color of their mother's hair or their first pet's name, their eye movements become a kind of map to the truth.

Most people look to one particular part of their brains to retrieve fact and a different part to create fiction. The eyes usually reflect these thought processes naturally. But be careful not to generalize the eye movements of one person for all people. Everyone is different. And really crafty people stare straight ahead all the time. You'll never be able to read them, so don't even try.

Let's say your boyfriend usually looks up and to the left when he's telling the truth. If you ask him if he's been sleeping around and he looks straight up, or up and to the right instead, you may have problems.

Manipulative? A little. Useful? Sometimes. Of course it's best to get things out in the open and establish trust without these kinds of parlor tricks, but when it comes to dealing with others, sometimes we need all the help we can get.

HOW TO MAKE EVERYONE THINK YOU'RE CHARMING AND FANTASTIC EVEN IF YOU AREN'T

The daughters of my parents' friends have all married successful chemists. They have their own houses and dogs and some of them are expecting babies. I like my parents' friends just fine, but I hate their daughters. And I cringe when conversations with these people turn to me. I think they mean well when they ask what I've been up to, what do I do for a living, am I seeing anyone, when am I going to get married, but it doesn't feel that way.

Instead, I'm reminded of the Japanese Christmas cake. My friend Heather explained that in Japan, if you're an unmarried woman older than twenty-five, you're considered a "Christmas cake." Christmas cakes are colorful, enticing, and tasty on or before Christmas day, but once the special day has passed, the cakes have lost their appeal. They are likely stale and crumbly, their icing smeared. They're on sale, and no one wants them. At first I thought this was just some quaint cultural difference, but somehow the idea that I'm officially a "spinster" started to get to me. For me, the Christmas cake concept is as powerful as it is ridiculous. When my parents' friends grill me about my personal life, I feel cakey and strange. They don't understand the life I've chosen for myself, and, frankly, I don't want them to. I only have to see these people about once a year (ironically, just after Christmastime), and I've managed to hit upon the perfect strategy.

Whether you're a Christmas cake or not, there's a way to survive uncomfortable social situations. The easiest way to make everyone think you're charming and fantastic is to ask all about them, then actually listen to what they have to say. You benefit a great deal from this strategy because you don't have to explain that you are working on a book called *The Lost Soul Companion* just now, or that your move to California was a disaster, and you learn all kinds of useful things in the process.

This works best when you start the conversation yourself but less so if they accosted you and got the first words in. Try extricating yourself from "So, what's your latest cause?" and you'll see what I mean.

That was exactly what Mr. Reed asked me right out of the gate at my family's New Year's Eve party. All I could think to say was, "Well, I listen to a lot of talk radio now . . . " Things would've been much better if I'd started the conversation myself, chock-full of tactful questions about Mr. Reed, his work, his pets, favorite books—anything but me. (As it was, I floundered around until I could fit in, "Enough about me. How in the name of Hell are you?")

This conversational style evolved from my old friend Scott's "I" exercise. Scott was always trying to improve his character, which, by the way, was already quite sturdy. He told me about the "I" exercise, and I've never forgotten it. He would see how long he could go without referring to himself in conversation. He avoided the first person entirely—no *I, me, my, mine* at all. I tried it too, but, as you can imagine, I didn't do nearly as well as he did. When I was successful at it, I noticed that I spoke at least half as much as usual and that I learned a great deal more than I normally would have about other people and events.

Try the "I" exercise when you find yourself cornered. It may seem artificial or forced at first, but with practice it can become second nature. Not to mention that the details of your private life are just that—private—and are reserved for just the right people. You get to keep yourself to yourself.

ANGER AND THE EVIL HEADS

I'm one of those people who rarely gets angry. That's not a source of pride; rather, it is a weakness of mine. There's something to be said for the occasional fit of rage—not for its effects on blood pressure, but for its incredible ability to motivate. Consider the gravel driveway incident.

I used to live out in the country in one half of a duplex. My landlady lived in the other half. It was a pretty good situation for a while, but one day she managed to infuriate me. (I don't even remember why. Such is the nature of anger . . .) She was a big lady, and her manner was somewhat intimidating, so I didn't feel comfortable picking any bones with her. Instead of calmly discussing my problem and then coming to some amicable solution, I did things my way.

We shared the long gravel driveway which led all the way up to our respective front doors. I knew exactly what I needed to do. I grabbed a big handful of gravel,

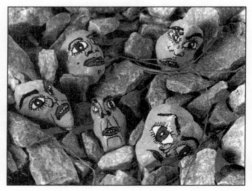

took it inside my part of the house, and proceeded to paint horrible little faces on the stones. The skin was very pink on each, the hair brown, and every face looked eerily like my landlady. With my technical pen, I detailed eyes and teeth and moles, then I sealed each little head with polyurethane. When every one was dry, I scooped them up, marched out to the driveway and tossed them all back. They landed in random spots, and I felt powerful simply because I knew they were there, leering up at my landlady as she got in and out of her minivan. This helped solidify my belief that if I couldn't be direct and polite while trying to resolve my anger with others, then I might as well try to get some good out of those negative feelings.

I was also reminded that karma is a boomerang. About three weeks after I released the evil heads into the landlady's driveway, I found them all together again, forming a circle near my entrance to the house. I was sure they were staring at me. I had brought them into the world, and now they were leering at me. I think the landlady must have been watching for me because she came right out, said she thought maybe I dropped some of my things, and, by the way, they were adorable. I mumbled my thanks, picked them up, and took them inside. You really do get what you give.

Something good did come of the evil heads, though. In some attempt to redeem myself, I turned the heads into kings and queens, bishops, knights, and pawns . . . I decoupaged a game board and turned my not-so-good deed into a chess set, which I then sold in order to pay my rent. It never hurts to channel your anger in some creative way. You may feel better and have something to show for your efforts too.

LIVING IN THE WORLD OF MEANIES

I don't need to tell you this, but there are some really horrible people in the world. People who want to see you fail. People who delight in your misfortune. You can do your best to treat others well, but, regardless, one of these days you're going to meet up with the human equivalent of napalm. I certainly have.

A company I worked for replaced a disgruntled employee with me. Soon after, I became the focus of his fury. He did everything in his power to discredit, humiliate, and undermine me. His attacks were public and personal. Worse yet, they have continued sporadically—even after the business closed! I carefully weighed my options at the time and finally decided what I should do about him—absolutely nothing.

No matter what, remember this: you can only have enemies if you allow yourself to have them. If someone tries to engage you in some miserable, bilious conflict, don't give such nonsense your time or energy. I realized that my life is too short to waste on my former coworker. You only have so long to offer your wonderful gifts to the people who deserve them, so don't waste your time on bad people.

That sounds simple enough, but it's very difficult to ignore those who want to hurt you. Still, you must. Here's why: they need your attention in order to thrive. Don't give it to them. Ignoring the meanies of the world gets easier with practice. It's difficult but not impossible. And it builds character like nothing else I know.

One thing that helped me to deal with my saboteur was to consider his motivation and point of view. Is someone out there trying desperately to hurt you? Maybe they're jealous of you and your talents or accomplishments. Perhaps you remind them of someone who abused them long ago. Whatever is behind their abominable behavior, you can be fairly certain that they are truly miserable inside. Think of them in compassionate terms and you'll feel too sorry for them to want to reciprocate with evil deeds of your own.

A WORD ABOUT COMPLETE STRANGER MEANIES . . .

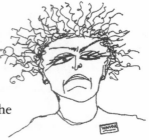

What about complete strangers who treat you badly? Give them the benefit of the doubt. When the lady at the grocery store checkout is surly with me, I say to myself, "Maybe her feet hurt." Negative energy is abundant in our world, and it spreads as quickly and easily as genital warts.

I'll never forget the time I was in my car, waiting to turn left at an intersection, when a middle-aged man wearing a business suit turned onto my street and stuck his tongue out at me as he rounded the turn. It was quite nasty and unexpected. As silly as it sounds, the incident upset me. I didn't even know him. What had I done to deserve that? I felt horrible for the rest of the day, and I had to resist the urge to pass the man's negative energy on to everyone else I encountered.

Spreading positive energy around takes more effort, but the effort is worthwhile. Try it and you'll understand what I mean.

GOOD MOVIES TO UPLIFT YOU

One of the best things to do when I feel hopeless and miserable is to escape with a movie. Every now and then it helps to forget my own difficulties for a time and get completely absorbed in someone else's—even if it is just smoke and mirrors.

These are some of the most original, uplifting movies I've ever seen. If you're feeling particularly dejected, maybe you'll like them.

- The Full Monty
- Good Will Hunting
- Say Anything
- Joe vs. the Volcano
- Breakfast at Tiffany's
- Cosi

THE ANTIBIOTIC MOVIES . . .

Antibiotic movies are the kind of movies that you have to watch from beginning to end if you are to enjoy their therapeutic effects. Like antibiotics, if you stop the course of treatment partway through, you'll have, in fact, done yourself more harm than good. So no matter what, you have to keep watching, even through the really terrible and sad parts. Be patient . . .

- Rushmore ← my all-time favorite!!!
- Dead Poets Society
- It's a Wonderful Life
- The Shawshank Redemption
- Scent of a Woman

BLOWING THE STINK OFF

Every now and then you just need to get out of the hole you're in. Get out of your room, out of your house, out of your town, and, as my dad says, "blow the stink off." There are some fantastic things to see and do in this world, and your time here is limited, so you might as well go exploring before your hips start to fail.

BURNING MAN

In August 1997, I packed up everything and moved with my then-boyfriend to Santa Cruz. In retrospect, I'd 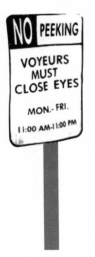 say the only good thing about moving from Indiana to California was stopping off at the Burning Man festival on the Hualapai Playa in Nevada along the way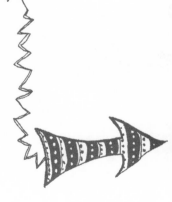

What is Burning Man?
(a little history...)

In 1986 a man named Larry Harvey built a human-like figure out of wood and burned it on a San Francisco beach. In honor of the summer solstice, 20 people came and watched the eight-foot construction burn. Since then, the figure—now called Burning Man—has increased in size and complexity. He's 50 feet of wood and metal and neon.

He's stuffed with explosives. Burning Man presides over a week long festival in the Nevada desert. The original crowd of 20 onlookers has now increased to about 15,000 active participants. Each year they bring enough food, water, and shelter to sustain themselves— and all kinds of artistic intangibles to share with everyone else. There are no spectators at Burning Man... just lots of impromptu theater, fashion shows, radio broadcasts, installations, and plenty of paradigm shifts.

I wouldn't have known about it at all if my boyfriend hadn't talked me into going, and, at first, I didn't like the idea too well. I thought it was some hippie fest, and I knew I wouldn't belong. Besides, I said, it was in the middle of Nowhere. What if something unthinkable happened?

Despite my qualms, we bumped over the playa in an enormous Ryder truck filled with everything we owned. The truth is, I felt very uncomfortable being officially homeless. He tried to tell me that I was home, that "home" was inside my own body. He wanted me to feel comfortable no matter where I was. (Although it was an estimable lesson, it didn't stick. To this day I quite like having an external, physical place to call home. A place with a sofa and a refrigerator and all my art supplies. A place where my doctor's phone number is always handy in case I freak out.)

But sometimes we have to take risks. I decided to accept the playa as my temporary home, and as it turned out, I never wanted to leave. The Black Rock Desert is 400 square miles of cracked, alkaline earth. During the Burning Man festival it's a weathered canvas and the thousands of people drawn to it are the paint. It's been said that people go to Burning Man to breathe art, and that is a perfect assessment.

How can I begin to explain just how blue the sky was? How the moon hung in the crisp desert dark? Have you ever jumped as high as you can on a trampoline at midnight under the biggest sky imaginable?

What struck me most about the festival was the sense of community, of belonging, of anything goes. For the first time in my life I discovered that the world is full of unusual, imaginative, kindhearted people. I wasn't as alone as I had thought I was.

Some fantastic bits

I met a woman who wore a bra made out of two sofa springs. She said it was much more comfortable than she thought

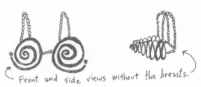

Front and side views without the breasts.

it would be—not to mention supportive. She was working at the BHOP—Barter House of Pancakes. I taught her my favorite magic tricks and she made me pancakes in exchange.

There were art cars everywhere! Most of which were simply indescribable. Some were even being made on the fly.

The human-powered bananamobile.

There was an old, boxy Lincoln completely covered with pennies. Understandably, the pennies had turned a beautiful green color near the wheel wells.

There were so many intriguing works of art, and most of them were burned. The joy is in their creation. Like Burning Man himself, their permanent, material existence is unessen-

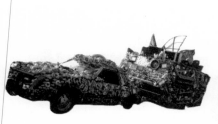

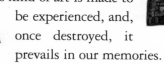

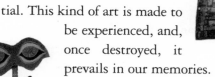

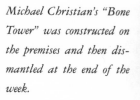

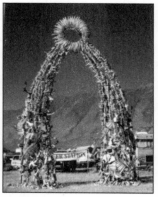

tial. This kind of art is made to be experienced, and, once destroyed, it prevails in our memories.

Michael Christian's "Bone Tower" was constructed on the premises and then dismantled at the end of the week.

Some of my favorite Burning Man camps: Bartertown, the Confessional of Conformity, Bianca's Smut Shack, and Crazy Dante's Used Soul Emporium. I can't—won't—begin to explain all of this. The Burning Man festival is just something you have to experience for yourself.

I did overhear some Burning Man veterans saying that the festival has gotten too commercial. That it was so

121

much better last year . . . But I'm reminded that any experience is only as good as you make it. Burning Man, for instance, is only as good for them as they allow it to be. The more I participated at Burning Man—and in life—the more involved and satisfied I felt.

At the end of the week it was time to burn the man. He had been an important landmark to me, and after he burned I was lost—literally. Without him towering over the makeshift community, I had trouble finding my way around. Not to mention how sad I was to see him go. I guess it was a good thing that it was time to move on.

I think the best part about traveling is coming "home." You almost always return a little bit changed—a little bit more than you were before you left.

ROAD TRIPPING

Don't think you'll make it to Burning Man anytime soon? That's OK. Lost Souls can find plenty of inspiration closer to home.

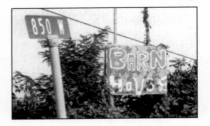

Just forty-five minutes from where I live, for instance, is the Barn House. Even though it's a little tricky to find, Jim

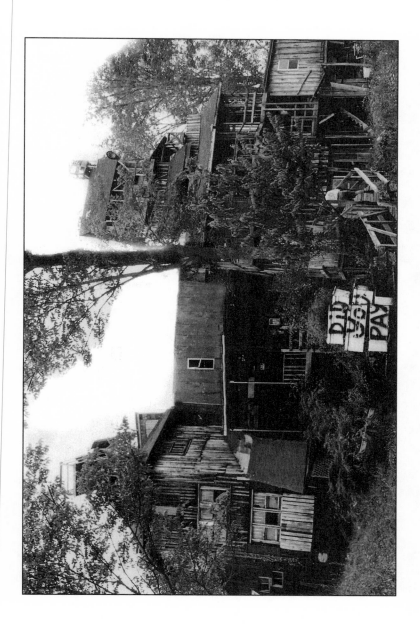

Pendleton's creation has attracted thousands of visitors from all over.

The Barn House is constructed from the remains of 11 houses and seven barns. It has 41 rooms, 100 feet of ladders, trapdoors, secret passages, two lookout towers, 15 stairways, and 15 decks. There are seven entryways in the front and seven more in back. It took Mr. Pendleton ten years to build. He used to live there with his family, but now he lives a few feet away in "Noah's Ark"—an upside-down ark designed to right itself when the floods come.

The view from the tallest tower in the Barn House is worth the terrifying climb up. Still, what impressed me the most was that one man thought up all of this and put it together with 1,800 pounds of nails and sheer will. The Barn House excursion taught me that there's no limit to what Lost Souls can accomplish if we want something badly enough. For now, *The Lost Soul Companion* project is my Barn House. What's yours?

If you have trouble finding your own local inspiration, try the *Roadside America* series by Mike Wilkins, Ken Smith, and Doug Kirby. They also have a very complete website at www.roadsideamerica.com.

PUCKITT THE ENCHANTED COCKATOO AND THE POWER OF PETS

I never used to pay much attention to birds. I thought only old people liked them. When I was younger my parents would point out the occasional hawk, but I was too cool to be bothered straining to see a dark speck in the sky.

Now I notice birds everywhere and I love them desperately. I know that they have tiny eyelashes and hollow bones, that they are resilient and magical creatures. Mostly that's because of Puckitt—my enchanted cockatoo.

Normally I wouldn't have chosen a bird for a pet. It seems wrong to keep them caged indoors when they could be out flying hundreds of feet up in the sky. I made an exception for Puckitt, because in his case the damage was already done.

My sister used to work in a pet store and she told me all about him. She said he was living with a family in West Virginia who didn't want him anymore. They'd kept him in a tiny cage crammed with other large birds for ten years and now, although he was reasonably healthy, he didn't seem quite right. So far no one would have him. Something clicked for me then. I was about to pay $300 for a parrot I'd never seen.

At first my parents tried to talk me out of it. Caring for a parrot—or any pet for that matter—is a big responsibility, and since I was in college, they reasoned, I didn't need anything else to take care of. I could, after all, barely take care of myself at the time and $300 was nearly all of my savings.

When I first saw him he had few feathers to speak of. He was wide-eyed and trembly and bald. I fell in love.

He was such a sweet creature. I didn't understand why anyone would keep him locked in a cage. Cockatoos and other parrots require as much love and attention as a typical two-year-old child. I got him used to the idea of being touched by holding him in a towel. He was frightened but very gentle. We worked together for a long time before I didn't need the towel anymore.

Focusing my energy and attention on Puckitt was very therapeutic for me. If I could make this creature more happy and comfortable, maybe I could do the same for myself someday.

Now I get up an hour early every morning just to snuggle with him, and I pet him for as long as he likes before I put him to bed. When I "bought" Puckitt, I thought I was just doing some good for a strange bird. As it turns out, he has done a great deal of good for me.

Puckitt comforts me. After his feathers grew back in, I

discovered that he's very absorbent. (I've been known to cry all over him and he doesn't seem to mind.)

He has even provided inspiration for several of my art exhibits.

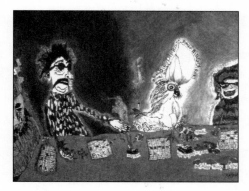

"Puckitt Wins Bingo" — detail from the very first in a long series of mixed media tributes to my friend...

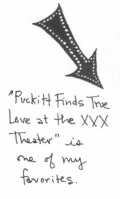

"Puckitt Finds True Love at the XXX Theater" is one of my favorites.

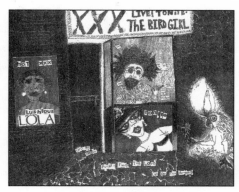

There are all kinds of creatures just like Puckitt who need good homes. Your local animal shelter is bursting with dogs and cats (and, yes, sometimes birds) who just had a bit of bad luck and are slated for the boneyard. If you're able to help one of them, you'll have helped yourself, too. Pets of the snuggly variety really can improve a Lost Soul's quality of life. (I count fish in with the non-snuggly variety. They can be very relaxing to watch, but that's not always enough.)

(Sorry fish!)

Dogs will exercise you regularly. Cats will demand you wake up at a decent hour each day. All snuggly pets remind their Lost Souls to be thankful for the little things.

4.

Living Well

LIFE IS A GIFT: EAT UP!

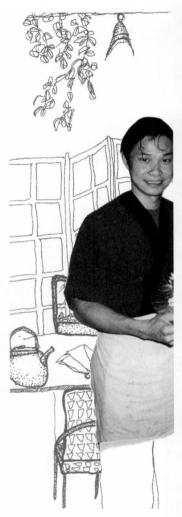

You never really know for sure what you have until it is gone. My friend Paul and I have a terrible weakness for sushi. Of all places to find fresh, expertly prepared sushi, Indiana should not readily spring to mind . . . and yet . . .

We lived in a college town that managed to support three sushi bars, but only one truly satisfied us. We really couldn't afford the place, but once in a while we decided to indulge.

The manager had a large, purple birthmark on his forehead. It crept over his left eye under his thick,

130

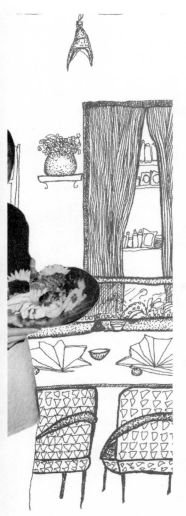

black-framed eyeglasses. He and Paul would chat about the stock market, and I would turn my attention to the chefs behind the long glass cases. One day I noticed someone new working behind the sushi bar. His name was Eddie and he had just arrived from New York to help out indefinitely. I knew preparing sushi and sashimi was an art form of sorts, but not until I met Eddie did I truly understand.

The other sushi chefs had always done an adequate job—our California rolls were carefully formed, the nigiri-style fingers of salmon and tuna neatly banded with deep green seaweed. But Eddie worked with a quiet intensity that I relished. He concentrated on every detail. Even the wasabi did not escape his attention. He carefully formed each bit of the spicy horseradish paste into the shape of a leaf—the surface of which he fin-

131

ished by drawing a few tiny veins with the tip of his knife.

Not long after we met him, he began to talk with Paul and me about his craft. He started making sushi when he was very young; it was something he always enjoyed. He shared some of the basics with us: the knife used to cut the rolls of fish and rice, for instance, should be wet at all times, and it is important not to cut against the grain of the rice. One day he asked us if we would like something special. Of course we would. It was the day Eddie made us our first green dragon.

I nearly cried when I saw it. The green dragon had salmon roe eyes, great, protruding whiskers, elaborate scales made out of thinly shaved avocado, and a neck band of seaweed. His segments were arranged so that he snaked around two exotic sauces in tiny silver cups. He was beautiful, and he was delicious. We ate him slowly and respectfully—the way one should eat any dragon.

Eddie photographed the green dragon, and the next time we visited him at the sushi bar, the photo—enlarged and laminated—was affixed to the restaurant window. We felt strangely flattered . . .

And there were other creations! Special dipping sauces, rolls made with fish skins, cucumbers turned into birds of paradise, even an arrangement he called the dreamboat. I wondered if he did this for everyone or just for us. And I asked myself, what would it be like to be his girlfriend and enjoy culinary pleasures reserved just for me?

It got to the point that we were going to the sushi bar a couple times every week, each of us spending upwards of $120 a month. There's only one thing that happened I'm still very sorry for, and it had nothing to do with the money. One day Paul, pagan that he is, wanted to have sushi and see a matinee in the same afternoon. I thought this was crazy; we would never have time to eat and make the movie that he hoped to see, but he wanted to try. We told Eddie about our plan, that we just wanted a quick fix. He whipped up some California rolls and a few other morsels, we devoured them and were gone in about ten minutes' time. I thought he looked disappointed that day, but I can't be sure. I told Paul we shouldn't have considered his art just a snack to inhale, but Paul thought I was being silly. It was, after all, a restaurant, he said.

A few months later Eddie left for good. He was going to Philadelphia to marry the girl he loved. The green dragon photo was taken down from the window since no one was able to make them like Eddie. We knew we were awfully lucky to have met him. You never really know what you have until it is gone. Appreciate what you have. Soon it may decide to move to Philadelphia.

Live Like You Have Cancer

What if you went to the doctor and he told you that you have metastasized, late-stage liver cancer? That you only had a few months to live? Your second and third and fourth opinions confirm the diagnosis, and even holistic healers shrug their shoulders. What then?

You decide to appreciate every last drop of your life. You find your way to New Zealand, eat great handfuls of candy in the middle of the night, make peace with your brother, try skydiving, pray, smoke Cuban cigars, stop telling lies . . . you do whatever it is you feel compelled to do.

And, just as you discover what is truly important, you also learn what not to spend your time and energy on. Working so many hours for somebody else just doesn't seem so important anymore. Neither does arguing with anyone about anything. And there is no time left for jealousy, greed, or hate.

For some people, being diagnosed with a terminal illness is one of the best things that ever happens to them.

What is it that you really long to do? You'd better do it because breathing in itself is a kind of terminal illness. We all know we're going to die—some of us even have a good idea of when—but do we really know how to live well?

While some amount of preparation for the future is still important, I try to live every day like I have cancer. I appreciate every minute as if it could be my last. And who knows? It could very well be.

BE THANKFUL YOU'RE NOT IN A TURKISH PRISON

Have you seen *Midnight Express*? It's an older movie directed by Alan Parker and it's based on a true story. This American guy tries to smuggle several kilos of hashish out of Turkey but gets caught and sent to a Turkish prison—and that's just in the first few minutes of the film! The prison is a filthy, torturous purgatory.

On the days when I am sitting in my cubicle at work hating my life and wishing I could just go home, I think to myself, "Well, at least you're not in a Turkish prison." I think back to the Turkish prison in *Midnight Express* with its dark stone walls and so much hopelessness. *Midnight Express* was just a movie, but we all know it represents a very real horror. At this very moment, someone is stuck in a Turkish prison. They may or may not be guilty of a crime, and they may never get out.

So what am I whining about? If I want to catch a bus, I can go out and catch a bus—to anywhere or nowhere in particular. If I want a great big piece of banana cream pie with meringue to the moon I can find one and devour it. My life is mine, and I am, for the most part, free free free.

Are you rotting away in a Turkish prison? I'm guessing not. That's one more blessing to count. Realize and relish your freedom. (Sometimes I forget . . .)

On Mailing Ridiculous Letters

A while ago I complained to my friend Paul that I lived a terribly dull life. He asked me what exactly made me think that my life was dull. I couldn't really put my finger on it. I told him I just knew everyone else had lots of friends. That they went to nightclubs and dinner parties. That they got mail. This last one got his attention. Mail? Yes, mail. I imagined that all people with exciting lives bounce over to their mailboxes every day, and they always find their boxes stuffed full of cards and packages with exotic markings. About two weeks later, Paul and I found a strange letter in my mailbox.

It was sent to my address, but the name on the envelope was Logan Marseilles. The previous tenant certainly was not called Logan Marseilles. There was no return address. Paul said I should open it, and I said no, I couldn't do that as the letter was clearly meant for someone else. But don't you want to open it? he asked. Well, sure, but . . . we can't. Well, maybe we could steam it open and then close it back again, I offered. At this, he rolled his eyes, snatched the letter out of my hands, and ripped it open with gusto. I clearly remember feeling shock and horror—mixed with delight. He handed me the naked letter. Paul said if you're going to do something, you might as well do it right, so I opened the epistle and began to read. Here's what it said:

Logan—

All is well on the front! I give daily offerings to the gods for the return of your health! You may, however, still contribute to our cause! You may no longer slay seven with one blow, but you may infiltrate the cursed corporation which prolongs our struggle through its financial dealings! Strike the beast in its heart! Sally your creative thoughts! I entrust the matter to your judgment and discretion! Now is the time to act!

> *Drive on!*
> *The Ambassador*

As I read it I glimpsed another world, another set of circumstances unfolding sometime, somewhere. It was a fantastic break from the life I knew. Never mind that Paul hadn't even bothered to disguise his handwriting. Forget that the letter made little sense and was punctuated almost entirely with exclamation marks. I really believed that I held something dangerous in my hands. I asked Paul if, perhaps, we should notify the police. I don't know how he was able to contain himself for so long, but he did. The hoax was delicious.

I used to know a man who wrote ridiculous letters to the TCBY yogurt people. It was a good hobby for him. There are a couple of very funny books by a man who calls himself Ted L. Nancy. *Letters from a Nut* and *More Letters from a Nut* are worth your time if you appreciate absurdity as much as I do. Try *The Lazlo Letters* by Don Novello, too. Maybe you'll be inspired to send ridiculous letters of your own. They're great diversions, and the world would be a better place if every mail carrier's satchel bulged with such playfulness.

MAKING WAVES

A few clever hoaxes and good-natured scams can greatly improve the quality of life for you and everyone around you. For instance, a long time ago my old friend Eric (a.k.a. Melva Small) submitted a fantastic recipe for "Fried Sugar Balls" to the "Neighbors" section of his local newspaper. On Monday, March 5, 1990, *The Herald-Times* gave Melva top honors by printing her submission under the heading "Recipe of the Week." Here it is, reprinted with permission of *The Herald-Times*:

Recipe of the week

Fried Sugar Balls

1½ cups granulated sugar

¼ cups powdered sugar

1½ cups lard

3 sticks margarine

Heat lard in skillet. Melt margarine, mix in granulated sugar and form balls, about 1-inch thick. Drop sugar balls into hot lard. Remove when golden brown. Serve hot on styrofoam plates, sprinkled generously with powdered sugar. This is a favorite of kids and grandparents alike. Even people who say they don't like lard like this dish.

Melva Small
Bloomington

Not long after the "recipe" came out, the newspaper ran a small piece explaining that they'd been had. Apparently a Brown County woman actually bought the ingredients, tried the recipe, and determined the dish was "unfit for human consumption." By May 7th, the recipe made its way to *The New Yorker* magazine. (Personally, I suspect Eric sent the clipping to the Big Apple himself—perhaps to breathe a little extra life into his well-crafted hoax.) *The New Yorker* printed the entire recipe and Melva's comments as they originally appeared in *The H-T*, including: "Even people who say they don't like lard like this dish." Folks at *The New Yorker* added: "If they live to tell the tale."

When I wanted to find and reprint this old recipe, I asked some of the old-timers at *The Herald-Times* if they knew how to make deep-fried sugar balls. You should have seen their faces light up! They all seemed delighted that they had been had by Melva Small so many years before.

I love this story because it's so absurd. Anything that wakes us up from the long sleep that our lives often become is a gift—even if it is disguised as a recipe for deep-fried sugar balls.

BE A PLAYFUL SOUL

My friend Benjamin is someone you just want to be around. He always seems to be up for anything. He is a playful soul.

In addition, he's drop-dead gorgeous. (I tease that he's hiding the Fountain of Youth under his sofa.) He has that indescribable movie star quality, but, actually, he's just Benjamin. He was once mistaken for Parker Stevenson from the *Hardy Boys* television series. And also for one of the Bay City Rollers. In both cases his "fans" simply would not leave him alone until they could get his autograph. He tried and tried to explain that he was, indeed, just Benjamin, but they wouldn't stand for it. Eventually he gave in. Smiling sheepishly, he signed autographs for them. Not only were they delighted that they ran into one of their favorite stars, but they were also extremely satisfied that they were able to press him into revealing his "true" identity. He's been mistaken for Bob Weir of the Grateful Dead, too (apparently there are similarities if Benjamin hasn't slept well), but, so far, no Bob Weir autographs have been required.

How well do you handle life's unusual situations? How would you react if a bunch of insatiable "fans" hounded you? Would you get freaked out and run away? Would you become exasperated and angry? In Benjamin's case, maybe the Universe wanted him to be a star, but, more likely, maybe it just wanted to see what he would do. I think any time you are given the opportunity to delight strangers you should take it. It's just good karma. I'm certain that good things happen to playful souls who open themselves up to spontaneity and fun.

GIVE AND GIVE AND GIVE UNTIL YOU (ALMOST) CAN'T GIVE ANY MORE

I used to be all sweetness and light. Really. I was so trusting, so giving, and so kind to everyone I saw. If I were to meet that little buttercup on the street today, I would, at the very least, bloody her nose. I would tell her to trust no one, to stop dating altogether, and to eat a little red meat once in a while. I'm sure I would make her cry.

Of course, the truth is, I miss her. No, I don't ever want to be that naive again, but I'd rather not continue to be this acrimonious either. Every day I try a little harder to remember what it was like to be that girl. She was willing to give to others—even people who mistreated her—unconditionally. Before the modern-me can murmur, "What a sap," I must stop myself and consider that, well, maybe that girl was on to something after all.

There's a lot to be said for giving of yourself to others, trusting people, showing your delicate underbelly a little more quickly than everyone else does. That sort of goodwill is, for the most part, contagious . . . even if it doesn't seem readily apparent. What is it about adulthood that makes us all forget this point? Watch children. Some of them have a thing or two to teach us.

In her book *Bird by Bird*, Anne Lamott bills the following as "the best true story on giving" that she knows of. It was told to her by Jack Kornfield of the Spirit Rock Meditation Center in Woodacre.

An eight-year-old boy had a younger sister who was dying of leukemia and he was told that without a blood transfusion she would die. His parents explained to him that his blood was probably compatible with hers, and if so, he could be the blood donor. They asked him if they could test his blood. He said sure. So they did, and it was a good match. Then they asked if he could give his sister a pint of blood, that it could be her only chance of living. He said he would have to think about it overnight.

The next day he went to his parents and said he was willing to donate the blood. So they took him to the hospital where he was put on a gurney beside his six-year-old sister. Both of them were hooked up to IVs. A nurse withdrew a pint of blood from the boy which was then put into the girl's IV. The boy lay on his gurney in silence while the blood dripped into his sister, until the doctor came over to see how he was doing. Then the boy opened his eyes and asked, "How soon until I start to die?"

Gifts of the Literal Sort

My friend Wes gave me a very special paper plate. It is one of the best gifts I've ever received.

A Paper Plate Story for Susan

Once there was a paper plate named Delores. Delores was the kind of paper plate that was kind of weak as paper plates go, the kind that required you use two lest your food soak through and leave a stain on your clothes. She came in a pack, an economy pack with 500 like plates. I say like plates, however from the beginning, Delores knew she was different from the others. People thought of her as a disposable plate, but we prefer to think that there is a right plate at the right time for everyone. The people who bought Delores immediately recognized that she was different (she had that certain special, undefinable <u>something</u>) and put her aside rather than eat on her. But Delores was a plate her purpose in life was to serve food. She knew that being used like this would just <u>feel</u> right. She was very sad to be singled out and not used. From her pack the plates were used in pairs so they'd be strong enough to contain big potluck meals, and the plates in the pack wished fervently that they'd be chosen as the top plate in a pair. Delores sat for some time up on top of the refrigerator feeling lonely and dejected. Then one day, someone looking for a piece of paper picked up and used Delores. She was rolled into the typewriter and was special, different and useful. Introducing Delores. Enchanter.

Things to always give: The benefit of the doubt, undivided attention, LOVE, the whole truth, Big Tips, kind words, joy, charm, encouragement, happiness, good deeds, laughter, hope. (These kinds of gifts are secretly gifts to ourselves...)

Things to Sometimes give: Constructive criticism, compliments, trust, affection, money.

ALWAYS, ALWAYS keep this: Your own power.

DAYDREAMS AND DOUBLE-DOG DARES

I dare you to imagine your own success. Are you a writer? Imagine yourself at your very own well-attended book signing. An artist? You've received great reviews and people have begun to collect your work. Are you a musician? You're signed to a respectable label, you're playing to full houses of appreciative fans. Let yourself dream from time to time. Letting your mind wander in these positive ways can help you to determine what it is you really want for yourself.

Of course dreaming in and of itself is virtually useless, but I'm sure you already know that. Daydreams combined with hard work and clever marketing will take you a very long way. The unpublished writer dreaming of well-attended book-signings can accomplish his goals by self-publishing his work and organizing his own book-signing tours. The lesser-known artist can organize his own art opening and hand deliver reception invitations to members of the press. Frustrated musicians can pool their resources, start their own record label, and sign themselves.

These may not seem like great strides, but you have to crawl before you walk. Typically, huge commercial success requires a lot of other people to buy into your work. Others are more likely to take a chance on you if you demonstrate dedication and believe in yourself. If you want something badly enough, you'll find a way to get it, and it may take a long time. A moment ago I dared you to imagine your own success. Now I double-dog dare you to accept that you have to start small.

THE WORM AMBULANCE

When I was eight I operated my own worm ambulance service. After every big rainstorm I used to take my brother's hot pink skateboard and my plastic bucket-and-shovel set and skate up and down our street saving rain-drenched worms from untimely deaths. If a worm had been partially smashed by a car I would cut his damaged piece away and toss the rest of him in the bucket with his friends. In a half hour I'd have an incredible collection of rescued worms!

When I was finished I would dump all of the worms out into what I believed was my garden. It was just a small patch of dirt in which I grew only carrots, since no other vegetable was worth eating at that time.

I still save drowning worms—only now I'm more discreet about it. And it's still extremely satisfying work. As the worm ambulance, I skated around with so much energy and determination. I really believed in what I was doing and I knew that I was just the right person for the job.

I hadn't felt that way about anything since then—until I began *The Lost Soul Companion.* Focusing my energy on helping other Lost Souls was the best thing I've done in a long time.

I've learned that Lost Souls who feel driven to do something constructive and good will succeed sooner or later.

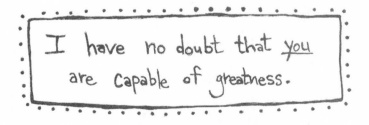

I have no doubt that _you_ are capable of greatness.

THE ENDING IS JUST THE BEGINNING

I am often sad when a book I've been reading ends. If you're sad that *this* book is over, please don't be. I didn't write it to make you sad!

You can find other Lost Souls and more support on my website: www.lostsoulcompanion.com

Or maybe you just want to correspond with me? Send an SASE to:

Lost Soul Companion Project
P.O. Box 3248
Bloomington, IN 47402-3248

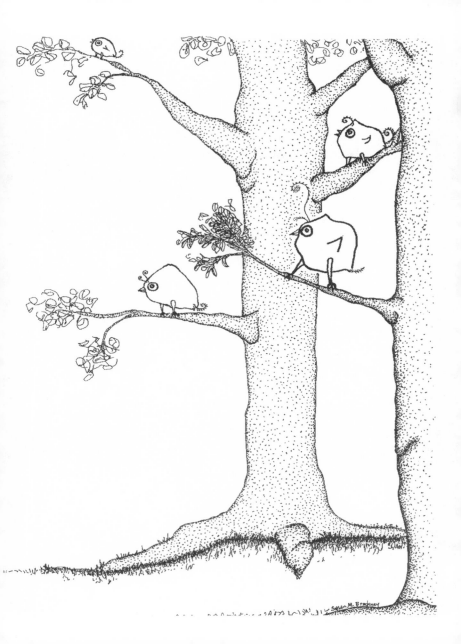

INDEX

153

154